Department of Veterans Affairs
Health Services Research & Development Service | Evidence-based Synthesis Program

Group Visits Focusing on Education for the Management of Chronic Conditions in Adults: A Systematic Review

December 2012

Prepared for:
Department of Veterans Affairs
Veterans Health Administration
Quality Enhancement Research Initiative (QUERI)
Health Services Research & Development Service
Washington, D.C. 20420

Prepared by:
Evidence-based Synthesis Program (ESP) Center
Portland VA Medical Center
Portland, OR
Devan Kansagara, M.D., M.C.R., Director

Investigators:
Principal Investigator:
Ana R. Quiñones, Ph.D., M.S.

Co-Investigators:
Jeannette Richardson, M.S.N., R.N., C.N.S.
Michele Freeman, M.P.H.
Maya E. O'Neil, Ph.D.
Devan Kansagara, M.D., M.C.R.

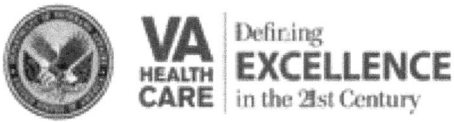

PREFACE

Quality Enhancement Research Initiative's (QUERI) Evidence-based Synthesis Program (ESP) was established to provide timely and accurate syntheses of targeted healthcare topics of particular importance to Veterans Affairs (VA) managers and policymakers, as they work to improve the health and healthcare of Veterans. The ESP disseminates these reports throughout VA.

QUERI provides funding for four ESP Centers and each Center has an active VA affiliation. The ESP Centers generate evidence syntheses on important clinical practice topics, and these reports help:
- develop clinical policies informed by evidence,
- guide the implementation of effective services to improve patient outcomes and to support VA clinical practice guidelines and performance measures, and
- set the direction for future research to address gaps in clinical knowledge.

In 2009, the ESP Coordinating Center was created to expand the capacity of QUERI Central Office and the four ESP sites by developing and maintaining program processes. In addition, the Center established a Steering Committee comprised of QUERI field-based investigators, VA Patient Care Services, Office of Quality and Performance, and Veterans Integrated Service Networks (VISN) Clinical Management Officers. The Steering Committee provides program oversight, guides strategic planning, coordinates dissemination activities, and develops collaborations with VA leadership to identify new ESP topics of importance to Veterans and the VA healthcare system.

Comments on this evidence report are welcome and can be sent to Nicole Floyd, ESP Coordinating Center Program Manager, at nicole.floyd@va.gov.

Recommended citation: Quiñones AR, Richardson J, Freeman M, O'Neil M, Kansagara D. Group Visits Focusing on Education for the Management of Chronic Conditions in Adults: A Systematic Review. VA-ESP Project #05-225; 2012

This report is based on research conducted by the Evidence-based Synthesis Program (ESP) Center located at the Portland VA Medical Center, Portland OR funded by the Department of Veterans Affairs, Veterans Health Administration, Office of Research and Development, Quality Enhancement Research Initiative. The findings and conclusions in this document are those of the author(s) who are responsible for its contents; the findings and conclusions do not necessarily represent the views of the Department of Veterans Affairs or the United States government. Therefore, no statement in this article should be construed as an official position of the Department of Veterans Affairs. No investigators have any affiliations or financial involvement (e.g., employment, consultancies, honoraria, stock ownership or options, expert testimony, grants or patents received or pending, or royalties) that conflict with material presented in the report

TABLE OF CONTENTS

Executive Summary
    Background 1
    Methods 2
    Results 2
    Discussion 6
    Conclusion 6

Introduction 7

Methods
    Topic Development 8
    Search Strategy 10
    Study Selection 10
    Data Abstraction 10
    Study Quality 11
    Rating the Body of Evidence 11
    Data Synthesis 11
    Peer Review 12

Results
    Literature Flow 13
    Findings by Key Question 15
        Key Question 1. In adults with chronic medical conditions, how do group visits compared to usual care affect the following: (1) medication adherence, biophysical markers (e.g., HbA1c, blood pressure); (2) symptom status, functional status, mortality, patient satisfaction; (3) utilization of medical resources, health care costs; (4) adverse outcomes (e.g., patient confidentiality, participation/missed appointments)? 15
        Key Question 2. For adults with chronic medical conditions, do the effects of group visits vary by patient characteristics? 15
        Key Question 3. Which components of group visits are associated with greater intervention effects? 16
    Findings by Clinical Area 16
        Arthritis 16
        History of Falls 17
        Asthma, COPD 24
        Hypertension, CHF, CAD 29
        Diabetes Mellitus 33
        Multiple Chronic Conditions 48
        Chronic Pain 51

Discussion 54
Generalizability 55
Limitations 56
Future Research 57
Conclusions 57

References 58

Tables

Table 1.	Characteristics of group visit interventions focusing on education for the management of arthritis or falls	18
Table 2.	Findings from interventions reporting standardized or validated measures that compare group visits to control, stratified by arthritis or falls	21
Table 3.	Summary of findings from head-to-head group visit interventions and group vs. individual visit interventions for patients with arthritis or falls	23
Table 4.	Characteristics of group visit interventions focusing on education for the management of asthma or COPD	25
Table 5.	Findings from interventions comparing group visits to usual care control for the management of Asthma or COPD, stratified by clinical area and outcome category	27
Table 6.	Summary of findings from head-to-head group visit interventions and group vs. individual visit interventions for patients with asthma or COPD	28
Table 7.	Characteristics of group visit interventions focusing on education for the management of congestive heart failure, coronary artery disease, or hypertension	30
Table 8.	Findings from interventions reporting standardized or validated measures that compare group visits to control, stratified by hypertension or CHF	32
Table 9.	Summary of findings from head-to-head group visit interventions and group vs. individual visit interventions for patients with hypertension or CHF	32
Table 10.	Characteristics of group visit interventions focusing on education for the management of diabetes mellitus	35
Table 11.	Findings from interventions reporting standardized or validated measures that compare group visits to usual care in the management of diabetes mellitus	40
Table 12.	Summary of findings from head-to-head group visit interventions and group vs. individual visit interventions for the management of diabetes mellitus	42
Table 13.	Characteristics of group visit interventions focusing on education for the management of chronic conditions in populations with multiple disease groups	49
Table 14.	Characteristics of group visit interventions focusing on education for the management of chronic conditions in populations with multiple disease groups	50
Table 15.	Characteristics of group visit interventions focusing on education for the management of chronic pain	52
Table 16.	Findings from interventions comparing group visits to control for the management of chronic pain	53
Table 17.	Findings from interventions comparing group visits to control for the management of chronic pain	53
Table 18.	Evidence gaps and future research	57

FIGURES

Figure 1.	Analytic framework to evaluate group visits	9
Figure 2.	Literature Flow	14
Figure 3.	Effect of group visits compared to usual care on HbA1C at ≤6 month follow-up, by study quality	44
Figure 4.	Effect of group visits on HbA1C compared to usual care at ≤6 month follow-up, by duration of intervention	45
Figure 5.	Effect of group visits compared to usual care on HbA1C at 7-12 month follow-up, by study quality	46
Figure 6.	Effect of group visits compared to usual care on HbA1C at 7-12 month follow-up, by duration of intervention	47

APPENDIX A.	SEARCH STRATEGY	67
APPENDIX B.	INCLUSION AND EXCLUSION CRITERIA	73
APPENDIX C.	QUALITY ASSESSMENT	75
Table C1.	Quality assessment and methodological characteristics of individual studies in randomized controlled trials of group visits	76
Table C2.	Total number of outcome measures reported in studies of group visit interventions focusing on education for the management of chronic disease	79
APPENDIX D.	PEER REVIEW COMMENTS AND RESPONSES	102
APPENDIX E.	GLOSSARY FOR OUTCOMES USED IN INCLUDED STUDIES	109

EXECUTIVE SUMMARY

BACKGROUND

The goal of group-based educational programs led by non-prescribing facilitators is to communicate information and provide training in order to improve self-management skills for the large numbers of patients coping with chronic illness. The Veterans Administration (VA) has prioritized group visit implementation as part a new primary care model that focuses on patient centeredness, The Patient Aligned Care Team (PACT), but the choice of which patient populations to target and which interventions to use is unclear. Though the group visit intervention delivery model has been widely used, there are vast differences in program structure, content, length of intervention, and follow-up time points. Moreover, there is little consensus as to whether, and for whom, group visits are an effective tool. Given the variety of interventions, the broad array of chronic conditions in which group visit interventions have been studied, and the lack of an overall understanding of effectiveness, it is useful to clarify what is known and not known about group visit interventions in patients with chronic illness. To our knowledge, no recent review has examined group visit interventions across a variety of conditions.

The objectives of this review are to: 1) summarize the characteristics of group visit interventions that have been tested in controlled trials of patients with chronic illness; 2) assess the effects of these interventions on quality of life, self-efficacy, health care utilization, and other health outcomes; 3) understand whether there are certain patient characteristics associated with intervention effectiveness; and 4) examine which components of group visit intervention structure and delivery may be associated with intervention effects.

We address three key questions in our review of the literature on group visits conducted by non-prescribing health professionals and lay facilitators:

Key Question 1. In adults with chronic medical conditions, how do group visits compared to usual care affect the following:

    (1) medication adherence, biophysical markers (e.g., HbA1c, blood pressure)

    (2) symptom status, functional status, mortality, patient satisfaction

    (3) utilization of medical resources, health care costs

    (4) adverse outcomes (e.g., patient confidentiality, participation/missed appointments)?

Key Question 2. For adults with chronic medical conditions, do the effects of group visits vary by patient characteristics? Characteristics of interest include medical diagnosis, severity of disease, and comorbidities.

Key Question 3. (Depending on the size and comparability of elements identified in the literature) Which components of group visits are associated with greater intervention effects?

METHODS

We conducted searches of multiple databases (MEDLINE® via PubMed®, Embase®, Cochrane Register of Controlled trials, CINAHL (EBSCO), PsycINFO) using terms for non-prescribing practitioners and group visit interventions, including but not limited to terms for group education, group program(me), group session(s). We obtained additional articles from systematic reviews, reference lists of pertinent studies, editorials, and by consulting experts. Reviewers trained in the critical analysis of literature assessed the titles and abstracts for relevance, and retrieved full-text articles for further review. We compiled a narrative synthesis of findings, highlighting studies that evaluated the effects of group visits, and describe the common characteristics and themes that emerged across studies and disease categories. We conducted meta-analyses of group visit trials for patients with diabetes for the mean difference in the change of HbA1c. We describe the overall quality of evidence for outcomes in each clinical subsection using a method developed by the GRADE Working Group.

RESULTS

We included 87 publications reporting on 81 group visit intervention studies focusing on education for the management of arthritis, falls prevention, asthma, chronic obstructive pulmonary disease, hypertension, congestive heart failure, diabetes mellitus, or chronic pain.

We examined findings by key question as well as by clinical area.

Findings by Key Question

Key Question 1. In adults with chronic medical conditions, how do group visits compared to usual care affect the following: (1) medication adherence, biophysical markers (e.g., HbA1c, blood pressure); (2) symptom status, functional status, mortality, patient satisfaction; (3) utilization of medical resources, health care costs; (4) adverse outcomes (e.g., patient confidentiality, participation/missed appointments)?

In general, group visit interventions in most clinical areas were associated with short- and medium-term improvements in self-efficacy; few studies examined longer-term outcomes. However, there was little evidence that interventions improved quality of life, functional status, or utilization outcomes. Group visit interventions were associated with modest short-term improvements in HbA1c, but the strength of this evidence was low because of inconsistent results across studies and methodological concerns in the studies finding the greatest benefit.

Key Question 2. For adults with chronic medical conditions, do the effects of group visits vary by patient characteristics?

Relatively few studies specifically examined how patient characteristics modified intervention effects. Overall, studies found little difference in group visit effectiveness according to patient demographic and socioeconomic characteristics. However, among studies of arthritis and history of falls, two studies found that obese patients tended to respond to aerobic exercise group visits more than participants with lower BMI on self-reported disability and falls. Among hypertension and heart failure studies, one study found patients with more years of education and better cognitive status showed greater short-term improvements in cardiac-specific quality of life. One chronic pain study noted that group visit effectiveness was modified by agency-orientation, with high agency-oriented participants experiencing improvements in pain and pain coping resulting from group visit sessions. Various authors note that small sample sizes limit the power to detect differences in subgroup analyses. In addition, findings of group visit benefit in subgroup analyses are tempered by fair and poor quality ratings for many of these studies.

Key Question 3. Which components of group visits are associated with greater intervention effects?

Overall, in five studies, group visit interventions that focused on self-management educational strategies were more effective than sessions that were limited to didactic education; however, in four of these five studies, the intervention arms differed considerably from the comparators (e.g., having nonequivalent number of sessions), limiting the strength of this conclusion. Studies that compared group visits to individual education visits found mixed results on a variety of outcomes, with no appreciable differences found in three studies, positive effects found with group visits in four other studies, and improvements with individual education in one study. Findings across studies could not be combined because of differences in study design. Two studies compared the effects of in-person group self-management education and mailed or automated self-management programs, and found no differences in self-efficacy, pain, and functional status outcomes.

Findings by Clinical Area

Arthritis

Eighteen studies from the US, Europe, and Australia evaluated the effectiveness of educational group visit interventions that included self-management skills (11 studies), didactic (8 studies), and experiential approaches (6 studies). Studies varied widely in intervention structure, content, and duration, as well as comparison group.

Seven of ten studies found group visit interventions improved short- and medium-term self-efficacy; six of the studies found benefit for the interventions focused on self-management skills education. Only one poor-quality study assessed outcomes beyond 12 months. Despite the improvements seen in self-efficacy, only two of eleven studies found improvements in quality of life related measures such as disability and depression. One US study found a self-management education intervention was associated with reduced physician visits, but this finding was not confirmed in five other studies conducted in Europe and Australia.

Overall, there is a moderately strong body of evidence that group self-management education interventions can improve short- and medium-term self-efficacy in patients with arthritis, but they have little effect on quality of life or utilization outcomes.

History of Falls

Four studies from the US, Canada, and Australia examine effectiveness of educational group visit interventions in patients with a history of falls or at-risk for falling. Overall, didactic falls prevention training along with exercise training may improve patient self-efficacy and reduce the risk of falls, though the strength of this evidence is low because of inconsistencies among studies and the small number of studies.

Asthma, COPD

Five studies conducted in the US or Australia examined the effects of group visit interventions compared with usual care in patients with asthma. The group interventions involved didactic education in four studies and self-management education in one study. Decreased utilization was observed in two studies, and improvements in quality of life measures were noted in two studies. The studies were limited by selection bias and other methodological issues, however, and study quality was generally poor.

Five studies of group visits in COPD patients were conducted in a variety of settings: Northern Ireland, the UK, the Netherlands, France, and a VA Medical Center in the US. Three studies compared didactic education combined with exercise training to didactic education alone or to usual care. Two other studies examined the effects of self-management education compared with didactic education, usual care, or individual support. Better exercise capacity was observed in the studies that combined exercise training with didactic education, as compared with usual care or with didactic education alone.

Overall, a small body of fair-to-good quality evidence suggests that group exercise training in combination with didactic education may be associated with small improvements or less decline over time in exercise capacity and COPD symptoms, though the clinical significance of these findings is unclear. There is little methodologically sound evidence examining the impact of group visits in patients with asthma.

Hypertension, CHF, CAD

Our literature search identified three fair-quality studies of group visit interventions conducted in patients with CHF or CAD, published in four reports. Six studies examined the effects of group visits on blood pressure in patients with hypertension. The studies were conducted in a range of international settings, and study quality varied widely. Three studies used self-management education techniques and two studies used didactic education in comparison with usual care or an informational control. One trial compared self-management education directly with didactic education. Reductions in blood pressure measurements were noted in all three self-management education studies and in one didactic education study. In the trial comparing self-management education directly with didactic education, there were no significant reductions in systolic or diastolic blood pressure in either group at three months. However, significantly more self-management education patients had controlled blood pressure.

Overall, there were very few studies of group visits in CHF patients, and their findings on self-efficacy, quality of life, and biophysical measures were largely neutral. Group self-management education interventions in patients with hypertension have reported improvements in blood pressure control in short-term and long-term studies, but the overall strength of evidence is low.

Diabetes Mellitus

We included 30 publications of 29 studies of group visit interventions in patients with diabetes mellitus. We conducted meta-analyses of the 17 studies comparing the effects of a group visit intervention to usual care on HbA1c. Overall, in 14 studies, group visit interventions reduced HbA1c slightly more over six months of follow-up than usual care, though there was significant heterogeneity which should temper confidence in these results. At least part of the heterogeneity seemed to be associated with study quality. The two good quality studies found no short-term improvements in HbA1c. Group visit interventions lasting more than three months appeared to have a more pronounced effect on HbA1c improvement than those of shorter duration, but the quality of these longer duration intervention studies was also lower. We found similar effects on HbA1c at 7 to 12 months in the 10 studies with longer-term follow-up.

Five of ten studies found improvements in self-efficacy or illness belief scores, with four of these studies finding positive effects beyond six months of follow-up. Perhaps not surprisingly, four of the five studies finding beneficial effects on self-efficacy involved interventions specifically focused on broader self-management skills training rather than didactic education. Despite finding that some interventions may improve self-efficacy, there was little evidence that group visit interventions improved quality of life over the short- or long-term. Few studies reported or were powered to evaluate utilization outcomes.

Eleven studies compared a group visit intervention to one or more active interventions. Three of these studies found that interventions focused on self-management skills training were associated with greater improvements in glycemic control than didactic educational approaches, though there were multiple other differences in the interventions being compared, making it difficult to draw firm conclusions about the effects of educational approach alone. Two studies compared group to individual education. One fair-quality study found that an automated, telephone-based, self-management intervention performed similarly to an in-person group self-management skills intervention.

Overall, we found group visit interventions in patients with diabetes may have modest effects on glycemic control over the short- and long-term, but the strength of evidence supporting this conclusion is low mostly because of inconsistencies across studies and methodological weaknesses of the studies finding the most positive effects. Interventions focused on self-management skills training were associated with improved self-efficacy and illness belief scores over the short- and long-term. However, there was no consistent evidence that group visit interventions improved quality of life.

Multiple Chronic Conditions

Four studies evaluated the Chronic Disease Self-Management Program (CDSMP) in populations with various chronic conditions not limited to a particular disease group. Overall, the peer-led, community-based CDSMP appears to be associated with medium-term improvements in self-efficacy, health status, and health care utilization; and these effects may persist long-term. These findings are based on moderately strong evidence from two large US trials, though findings were not replicated in other countries, and the findings likely apply most to patients engaged enough in care to agree to attend a multi-week course.

Chronic Pain

Four studies evaluated the effects of group-based interventions compared to usual care, educational reading materials, or individual treatment in patients with chronic pain. Though many findings from the studies were not statistically significant and did not differ from the comparison, some results favored the group-based interventions. Overall, a very small body of literature suggests group-based, self-management education interventions may improve pain coping skills at least over the short-term, though the strength of this evidence is low because there were few studies and the methodological quality of one of the studies finding benefit was poor.

DISCUSSION

We found 79 trials examining the effects of group visit interventions across a variety of chronic illnesses. Despite the large evidence base, it is difficult to draw overall conclusions about the effectiveness of group visit interventions in patients with chronic illness, in part because of the diversity of patient populations studied, interventions tested and outcomes reported. Nevertheless, in general, many group visit interventions appear to be able to improve short- and medium-term patient self-efficacy, but there was little consistent, fair-to-good quality evidence that they improved quality of life, health outcomes, or health care utilization. We found that diabetes group visit interventions were likely associated with small short-term improvements in glycemic control. The longer-term effects of group visit interventions are largely unknown since the vast majority of studies focused on short-term effects.

CONCLUSION

Whether group visit expenditures are warranted may depend on how highly more proximate outcome measures like self-efficacy are valued by patients and the health system. On the other hand, peer-led, community-based self-management programs are a low-cost intervention which appears to improve self-efficacy and, in mixed groups of patients with various chronic illnesses, may improve health and utilization outcomes. Group visits may be as effective as individual education visits and may represent a reasonable alternative for educating patients with chronic illness, though the varied and sometimes low participation and retention rates suggest they should not be the sole alternative.

Return to Contents

EVIDENCE REPORT

INTRODUCTION

The goal of group-based educational programs led by non-prescribing practitioners is to communicate information and provide training in order to improve self-management skills for the large numbers of patients coping with chronic illness. The Veterans Administration (VA) has prioritized group visit implementation as part of a new primary care model that focuses on patient centeredness, The Patient Aligned Care Team (PACT), but the choice of which patient populations to target and which interventions to use is unclear. Though the group visit intervention delivery model has been widely used there are vast differences in program structure, content, length of intervention, and follow-up time points. Moreover, there is little consensus as to whether, and for whom, group visits are an effective tool. Given the variety of interventions, the broad array of chronic conditions in which group visit interventions have been studied, and the lack of an overall understanding of effectiveness, it is useful to clarify what is known and not known about group visit interventions in patients with chronic illness. To our knowledge, no recent review has examined group visit interventions across a variety of conditions.

The objectives of this review are to: 1) summarize the characteristics of group visit interventions that have been tested in controlled trials of patients with chronic illness; 2) assess the effects of these interventions on quality of life, self-efficacy, health care utilization, and other health outcomes; 3) understand whether there are certain patient characteristics associated with intervention effectiveness; and 4) examine which components of group visit intervention structure and delivery may be associated with intervention effects. This review serves as a companion piece to the recently published shared medical appointments review conducted by the Durham Evidence-based Synthesis Program.[1] The shared medical appointments review focuses on visits led by a physician or other prescribing provider during which individual-level changes in management plan can be made. This review, in contrast, focuses exclusively on literature that tests the effectiveness of group visits that have an emphasis on health education and are led by facilitators, including but not limited to non-prescribing health professionals such as nurses, dietitians, and physical therapists.

Return to Contents

METHODS

TOPIC DEVELOPMENT

The review was commissioned by the Department of Veterans Affairs' Evidence-based Synthesis Program. We conferred with VA experts to refine selection of patient populations and subgroups, interventions, outcomes, and setting addressed in the review. The current review focuses on studies involving education-based group visits interventions led by facilitators that include non-prescribing health professionals.

We addressed the following key questions in our review of the literature:

Key Question 1. In adults with chronic medical conditions, how do group visits compared to usual care affect the following:

    (1) medication adherence, biophysical markers (e.g., HbA1c, blood pressure)
    (2) symptom status, functional status, mortality, patient satisfaction
    (3) utilization of medical resources, health care costs
    (4) adverse outcomes (e.g., patient confidentiality, participation/missed appointments)?

Key Question 2. For adults with chronic medical conditions, do the effects of group visits vary by patient characteristics? Characteristics of interest include medical diagnosis, severity of disease, and comorbidities.

Key Question 3. (Depending on the size and comparability of elements identified in the literature) Which components of group visits are associated with greater intervention effects?

The criteria for patient population, treatment and comparator interventions, outcomes of interest, and patient care setting are outlined below:

- **Patients**: Diagnosed with DM, HTN, CHF, COPD, asthma, arthritis, pain management, history of falls. Exclude comorbid serious mental illness such as schizophrenia. Studies with patients who have comorbid depression may be included.
- **Intervention**: Group visits focusing on education that are led by individuals who are non-prescribing health professionals as well as lay facilitators (e.g., dietitians, nurses, social workers, peer educators, psychologists, pulmonary technicians, physical therapists, occupational therapists). Group visits may include prescribing providers (e.g., physicians, pharmacists, advanced practice nurses, physician assistants) if they function in an advisory capacity only (i.e., do not provide individual care plans or medication management).
- **Comparator**: Usual care, non-group visit care
- **Outcome**: Biophysical/physiological (e.g., HbA1c, blood pressure) control of these markers/measures, rehospitalizations, medication adherence, ED visits, functional status, patient satisfaction, patient participation, and attrition rates.
- **Timing**: Any
- **Setting**: Any

Figure 1 illustrates the analytic framework that guided our review and synthesis.

Group Visits Focusing on Education for the Management of Chronic Conditions in Adults

Figure 1. Analytic framework to evaluate group visits

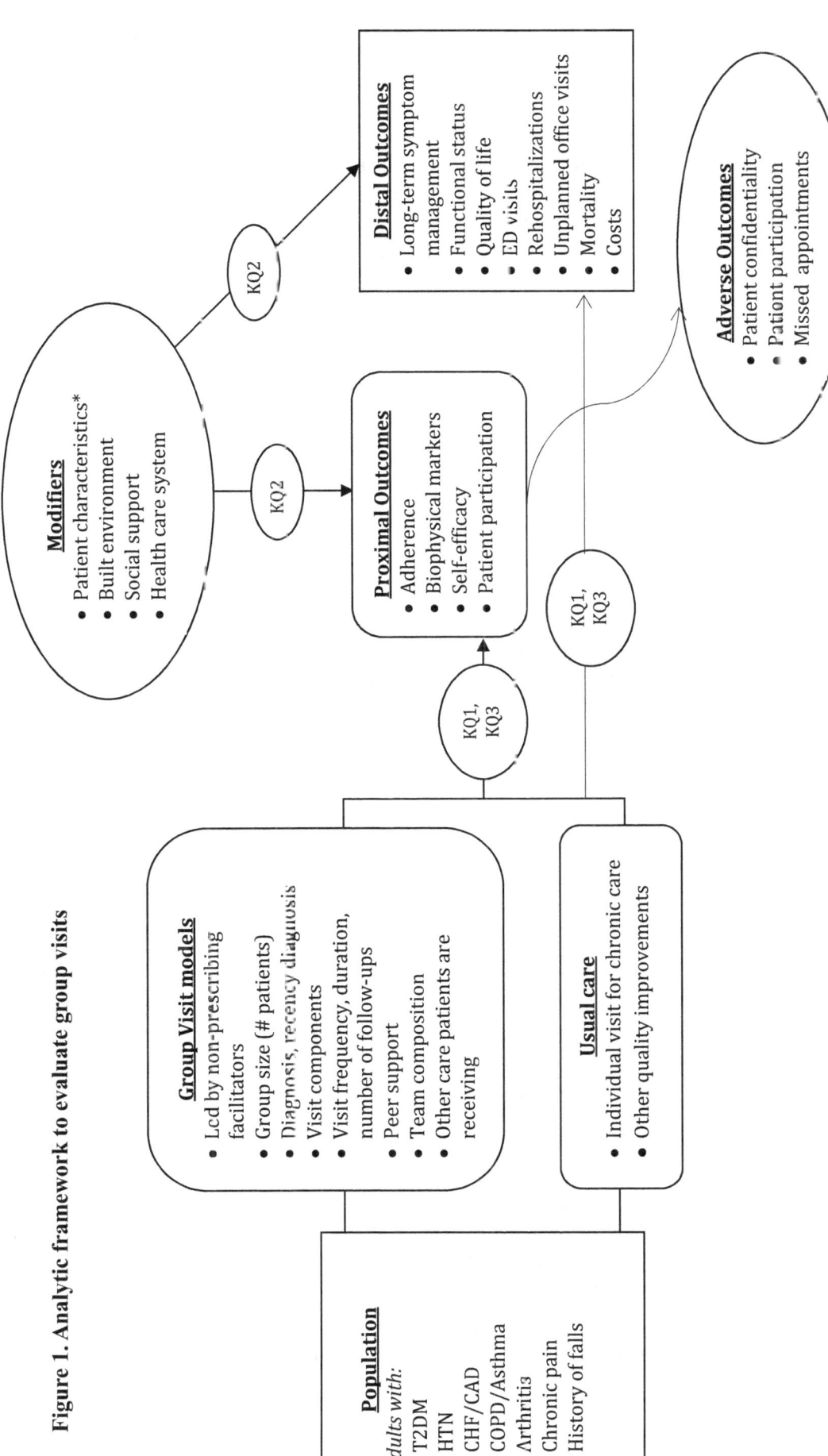

* Includes: gender, race/ethnicity, age, education/health literacy, rurality/geography, chronic conditions/morbidity, and other patient demographics. Note: socioeconomic influences such as financial strain (e.g., price of gas) directly affect patient participation

SEARCH STRATEGY

We conducted searches of multiple databases [MEDLINE® (PubMed®), Embase® (Embase.com), Cochrane Register of Controlled Trials (Ovid), CINAHL (EBSCO) and PsycINFO (Ovid)] from database inception to February 2012 using terms for non-prescribing practitioners and group visit interventions, including but not limited to terms for group education, group program(me), group session(s). See Appendix A for the full search strategy. We obtained additional articles from systematic reviews, reference lists of pertinent studies, editorials, and by consulting experts.

STUDY SELECTION

Reviewers trained in the critical analysis of literature assessed the titles and abstracts for relevance. Two investigators (AQ, JR, MF, MO, or DK) independently evaluated English-language articles included at the abstract stage using prespecified inclusion criteria (Appendix B). We included studies of group visit educational interventions led by non-prescribing facilitators. We excluded group visit studies if any portion of the intervention focused on individual-level prescription changes (e.g., blood pressure medication or insulin titration). We did not examine studies that focused exclusively on support groups or on group exercise classes (e.g., yoga, aerobic exercise, resistance training) without incorporating disease-pertinent educational components or comparing these interventions to group educational sessions. Existing Cochrane reviews of group exercise summarize the effectiveness of these interventions and represent a systematic evaluation of that literature.[2,3] We excluded diabetes mellitus studies published before 1998 because we felt the overall approach to adult diabetes care was likely to have changed substantially after publication of the United Kingdom Prospective Diabetes Study, thereby rendering older studies less directly applicable today.[4]

DATA ABSTRACTION

We abstracted data on the design, objectives, setting, population, demographics, findings, structure of the intervention, information on the comparator(s), and participation and attrition rates that characterized included studies. We also abstracted information on the content delivered in the group visit interventions. We distinguished between group visits whose content was to provide didactic-only educational sessions, and those that provided participants with information and training on techniques to improve coping and self-management skills. We defined the following, and abstracted this information from included studies:

- **Self-management education (SME):** In addition to providing disease-specific information to patients, these programs teach patients self-management skills to manage/cope with symptoms, such as goal-setting and contracting, and building skills to reinterpret symptoms (e.g., motivational interviewing, goal-setting/contracting, cognitive behavioral therapy (CBT))
- **Didactic education (DE):** Content is informational and format is usually lecture-based (e.g., information on the pathophysiology of disease, symptoms, using and reading equipment, potential strategies for reducing pain and stress, understanding nutritional advice)
- **Experiential education (EE):** Instruction based on demonstrations (e.g., exercise, cooking, reading nutritional labels and calculating nutritional information)

STUDY QUALITY

Two reviewers independently assessed the quality of each trial according to the following criteria: randomization, allocation concealment, blinding and outcome reporting, as well as considerations for similarity of compared groups at baseline, adequate reporting of participation, loss to follow-up and attrition, the use of intention-to-treat analysis; and ascertainment of outcomes.[5] Individual studies were rated as "good," "fair," or "poor"; these terms are defined in Appendix C.

RATING THE BODY OF EVIDENCE

We describe the overall quality of evidence for outcomes in each clinical subsection using a method developed by the GRADE Working Group.[6] The GRADE method considers the consistency, coherence, and applicability of a body of evidence, as well as the internal validity of individual studies, to classify the grade of evidence across outcomes as follows:

- High = Further research is very unlikely to change our confidence on the estimate of effect.
- Moderate = Further research is likely to have an important impact on our confidence in the estimate of effect and may change the estimate.
- Low = Further research is very likely to have an important impact on our confidence in the estimate of effect and is likely to change the estimate.
- Very Low = Any estimate of effect is very uncertain.

DATA SYNTHESIS

During an initial informal review of included studies, we recognized that there was a breadth of outcome categories examined, marked variation in outcome metric validity, and a large number of different outcomes measured and reported across studies. We anticipated such challenges would render a full accounting and synthesis of all outcomes both infeasible and uninformative. We chose, therefore, to focus on distal health outcomes measuring quality of life and functional status because these are likely to be important to patients and could conceivably be impacted by the interventions examined in the studies under consideration. We included utilization outcomes when reported, though we anticipated that fewer studies would be powered to examine these outcomes. We also examined intermediate outcome metrics, focusing specifically on biophysical markers such as hemoglobin A1c, and on self-efficacy or patient activation measures. Self-efficacy refers to personal beliefs in one's ability to succeed in self-managing illness. In this report, we used the term broadly and used it to refer to any measures examining self-efficacy, patient activation, coping skills, or illness beliefs. We chose to examine this group of outcomes because there are validated tools to assess self-efficacy related concepts,[7,8] and these metrics were commonly reported in many studies. Furthermore, there is a link, both conceptually and empirically, between the knowledge, skills, and attitude changes one might acquire during an educational intervention and intermediate health outcomes.[9]

In compiling data tables, we prioritized well-validated scales and if studies report findings for full scales as well as subscales, we report full scales only. If studies did not report any outcome in these categories, or report ad-hoc/non-validated measures, their findings were summarized narratively. We also described common characteristics and themes that emerged across studies and disease categories.

We conducted meta-analyses of group visit trials for patients with diabetes for the mean difference in the change of HbA1c because we identified HbA1c as a clinically important marker for diabetes patients and one that is plausibly amenable to change in the short (0-3 months) and medium (4-6 months) term. We abstracted the mean difference and an indicator for variability (e.g., standard error) in HbA1c, and total subjects from each treatment arm. We obtained a pooled estimate of relative risk (RR) using a random effects model.[10] To determine whether the effects of group visits were modified by intervention characteristics, we conducted subanalyses according to study quality, and duration of the group visit intervention.

Statistical heterogeneity was assessed by Cochran's Q test and I^2 statistic.[11] In order to examine publication bias, we used funnel plots and Egger's test to assess small study effects.[12] We also conducted multivariate meta-regression analyses to determine whether duration of intervention, study quality, or publication year had any bearing on meta-analytic results. All analyses were performed using Stata 10.0 (StataCorp, College Station, TX, 2007).

PEER REVIEW

A draft version of this report was sent to the technical expert panel and additional peer reviewers. Appendix D details the feedback we received and our responses to reviewer comments.

RESULTS

LITERATURE FLOW

We reviewed 2,493 titles and abstracts from the electronic search, and identified an additional 42 studies from reviewing reference lists. After applying inclusion/exclusion criteria at the abstract level, 599 full-text articles were reviewed, as shown in Figure 1. Of the full-text articles, we excluded 512 that did not meet inclusion criteria.

We included 87 publications reporting on 81 group visit intervention studies focusing on education for the management of arthritis, falls prevention, asthma, COPD, hypertension, CHF/CAD, DM, or chronic pain. Tables 1, 4, 7, 10, 13, and 15 present characteristics of group visit interventions. Tables 3, 6, 9, 12, and 17 present head-to-head comparisons of multiple active group visit treatment arms as well as studies that compared individual visits to group visits.

Figure 2. Literature Flow – Group visits focusing on education for the management of chronic conditions in adults: A systematic review

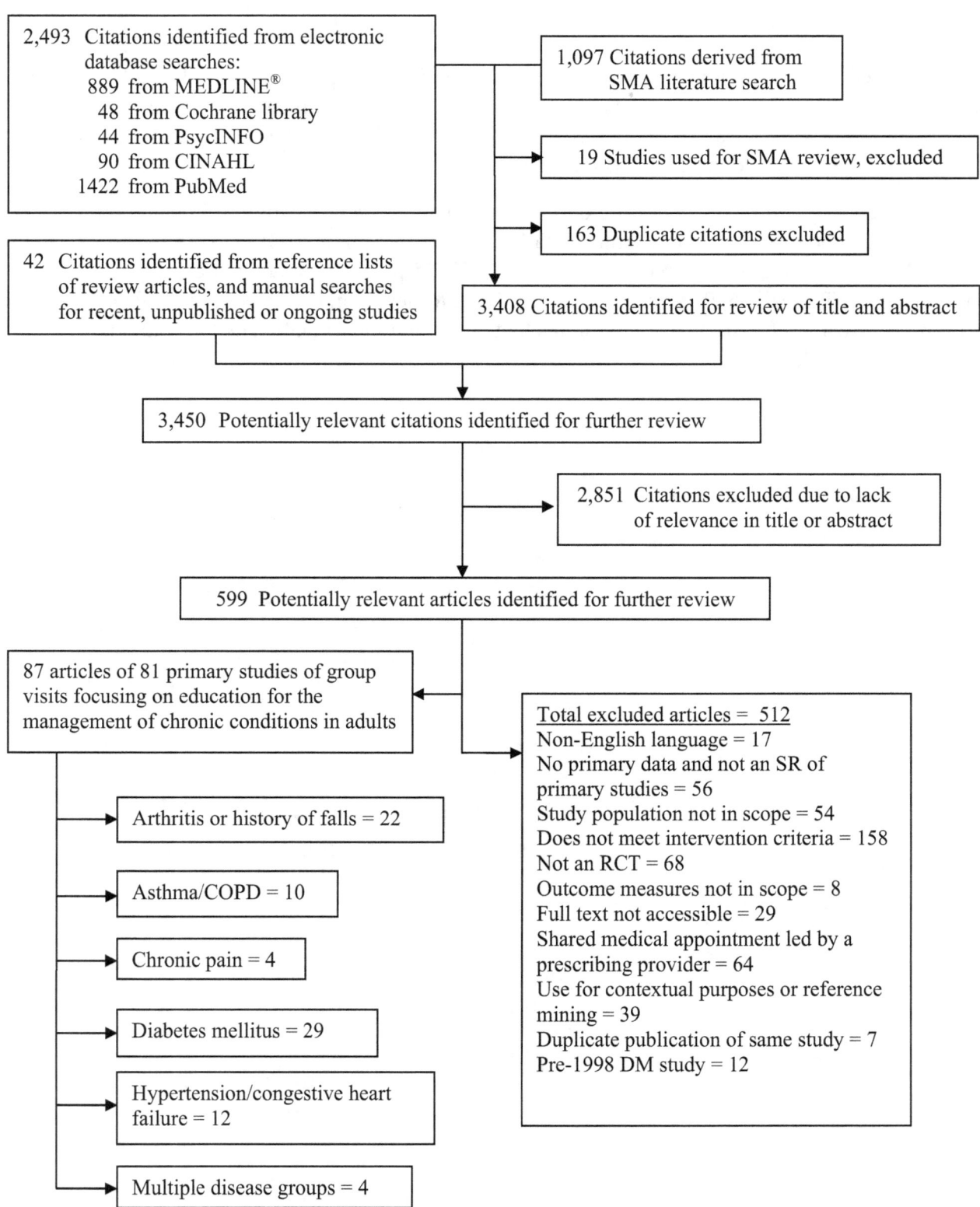

Findings by Key Question

Key Question 1: In adults with chronic medical conditions, how do group visits compared to usual care affect the following: (1) medication adherence, biophysical markers; (2) symptom status, functional status, mortality, patient satisfaction; (3) utilization of medical resources, health care costs; (4) adverse outcomes?

Tables 2, 5, 8, 11, 14, and 16 present findings of effectiveness of group visit interventions compared to usual care in the short (0-3 months), medium (4-6 months), long-term (7-12 months), or very long-term (13+ months). In addition, we present a full accounting of the total number of outcomes examined by studies in Appendix Table C2. Appendix E provides a glossary of acronyms and abbreviations for outcomes used in the included studies. We present findings from meta-analyses of mean change in HbA1c following group visit intervention for patients with diabetes mellitus in Figures 3 to 6.

Overall, group visit interventions in most clinical areas were associated with short- and medium-term improvements in self-efficacy; few studies examining longer-term outcomes. However, there was little evidence that interventions improved quality of life, functional status, or utilization outcomes. Group visit interventions were associated with modest short-term improvements in HbA1c, but the strength of this evidence was low because of inconsistent results across studies and methodological concerns in the studies finding the greatest benefit.

Key Question 2: For adults with chronic medical conditions, do the effects of group visits vary by patient characteristics?

Relatively few studies specifically examined how patient characteristics modified intervention effects. Sixteen studies presented results of group visit interventions by patient characteristics: nine diabetes mellitus studies,[13-21] two arthritis studies,[22,23] two history of falls studies,[24,25] one hypertension study,[26] one CHF study,[27] and one chronic pain study.[28]

Many of these studies examined group visit effectiveness for participants who attended a greater number of sessions relative to those with greater absentee rates.[13,16,18,19] Overall, the studies found some indications of a dose-response with group session attendance, with those participants attending the greatest number of sessions benefitting the most from the group visit intervention. For the DM studies, many found larger beneficial group visit intervention effects for patients with higher initial levels of HbA1c.[14,17,21]

Overall, studies found little difference in group visit effectiveness according to patient demographic and socioeconomic characteristics (e.g., gender, education, age, race). However, among studies of arthritis and history of falls, two studies found that obese patients tended to respond to aerobic exercise group visits more than participants with lower BMI on self-reported disability[22] and falls.[24] Among hypertension and CHF studies, Smeulders et al. found patients with more years of education and better cognitive status showed greater short-term improvements in cardiac-specific QoL.[27] One chronic pain study noted that group visit effectiveness was modified by agency-orientation, with high agency-oriented participants experiencing improvements in pain and pain coping resulting from group visit sessions.[28]

Various authors note that small sample sizes limit the power to detect differences in subgroup analyses. In addition, findings of group visit benefit in subgroup analyses are tempered by fair and poor quality ratings for many of these studies.

Key Question 3: Which components of group visits are associated with greater intervention effects?

Tables 3, 6, 9, 12, and 17 present findings of effectiveness of group visit interventions from head-to-head comparisons of multiple active group visit treatment arms, as well as studies that compared individual visits to group visits. Overall, in five studies, group visit interventions that focused on SME strategies were more effective than sessions that were limited to DE; however, in four of these five studies, the intervention arms differed considerably from the comparators (e.g., having nonequivalent number of sessions), limiting the strength of this conclusion. Studies that compared group visits to individual education visits found mixed results on a variety of outcomes, with no appreciable differences found in three studies, positive effects found with group visits in four other studies, and improvements with individual education in one study. Findings across studies could not be combined because of differences in study design. Two studies compared the effects of in-person group SME and mailed or automated self-management programs, and found no differences in self-efficacy, pain, and functional status outcomes.[29,30]

Findings by Clinical Area

Arthritis

Eighteen studies from the US, Europe, and Australia evaluated the effectiveness of educational group visit interventions that included self-management skills (eleven studies), didactic (eight studies), and experiential approaches (six studies).[22,23,29,31-44] Studies varied widely in intervention structure, content, and duration, as well as comparison group (Tables 1-3).

Seven of ten studies found group visit interventions improved short- and medium-term self-efficacy; in six of the studies finding benefit the interventions focused on self-management skills education. Only one poor-quality study assessed outcomes beyond 12 months.[44] Despite the improvements seen in self-efficacy, only two of eleven studies found improvements in quality of life related measures such as disability[41] and depression.[32] One US study found a self-management education intervention was associated with reduced physician visits,[41] but this finding was not confirmed in five other studies conducted in Europe and Australia.[31,32,34,35,40]

Eight studies compared two active interventions (Table 3). Many of these studies were comparing interventions with more than one characteristic that differed (i.e., different educational content and different number of sessions), making it more difficult to assess which intervention components may have been associated with observed effects. One study compared a self-management to a didactic education intervention with the same number of sessions and found no difference in outcomes between them.[36] Another study found that the inclusion of significant others along with patients in a self-management education intervention was actually associated with lower self-efficacy than the intervention delivered to patients alone.[42] Finally, one study found similar effects from a mail-delivered individualized self-management program and an in-person group self-management education intervention.[29]

Overall, there is a moderately strong body of evidence that group self-management education interventions can improve short- and medium-term self-efficacy in patients with arthritis, but they have little effect on quality of life or utilization outcomes.

History of Falls

Four studies from the US, Canada, and Australia examine effectiveness of educational group visit interventions in patients with a history of falls or at-risk for falling (Tables 1-3).[24,25,45,46]

Two studies found a group didactic education and exercise intervention improved self-efficacy over the short-term,[45] while another study which included a "booster" education session at three months found improved long-term self-efficacy.[24] One study found improved timed-up-and-go (TUG) physical performance,[24] while another study found the intervention did not improve TUG when patients were simultaneously tasked with cognitive activities.[25] Only one of three studies found a reduction in fall events,[24] and no studies found improved quality of life.

Overall, didactic falls prevention training along with exercise training may improve patient self-efficacy and reduce the risk of falls, though the strength of this evidence is low because of inconsistencies among studies and the small number of studies.

Group Visits Focusing on Education for the Management of Chronic Conditions in Adults

Table 1. Characteristics of group visit interventions focusing on education for the management of arthritis or falls

Study	Sample size Setting Program name, if applicable	Demographics: Mean age % male % minority Mean disease duration	GV structure: # Visits, frequency Duration Group size	GV content: SME (self-mgmt) DE (didactic) EE (experiential)	GV leaders: Number of leaders Profession type	Comparator(s)
Arthritis						
Ackerman, 2012[31]	N=120 Australia *ASMP*	65.1 yrs 40% Race NR Duration NR	6 weekly (2h) sessions 1.5 months 4-21 patients	SME	2 leaders Peer leader, health professional	Usual care (information book)
Barlow, 2000[32]	N=544 UK *ASMP*	58.1 yrs 16% 4% nonwhite 11 yrs with arthritis	6 weekly (2h) sessions 1.5 months ≥10 patients	SME	2 leaders Peer leaders	Usual care
Breedland, 2011[33]	N=34 Netherlands *FIT*	48 yrs 29% Race NR 9.7 yrs with RA	8 weekly (1h) education 16 semi-weekly (1.5h) exercise 2 months Group size NR	DE, EE	5 team members Psychologist, PT, OT, dietitian, social worker	Usual care
Buszewicz, 2006[34] & Patel, 2009[35]	N=812 UK *ASMP*	68.6 yrs 37% 0.5% Caribbean black Duration NR	6 weekly (2.5h) sessions 1.5 months 12-18 patients	SME, EE	NR	Usual care (information book)
Ettinger, 1997[22]	N=439 US *FAST*	69 yrs 30% 26% black Duration NR	3 monthly (1.5h) sessions 18 biweekly and monthly calls 18 months 10-15 patients	DE	2 leaders Exercise leader, nurse	Group exercise arms: GV2: 36 (1h) aerobic GV3: 36 (1h) resistance Class sizes 10-15
Freeman, 2002[36]	N=54 UK	51.4 yrs 15% Race NR 4.5 months with RA	4 weekly (2h) sessions 1 month Group size NR	GV1: SME GV2: DE	3 team members Physiotherapist, rheumatologist, psychologist	GV2
Giraudet-Le Quintrec, 2007[37]	N=208 France	54.8 yrs 14.1% Race NR 13.1 yrs with RA	8 weekly (6h) sessions 1 (4h) booster after 6 months 2 months 8-10 patients	DE, EE	10 team members Rheumatologist, rehab. specialist, dietitian, social assist., nurses, PTs, and OTs	Usual care+: Two information leaflets written by research team
Hammond, 1999[23]	N=35 UK	55.2 yrs 17% Race NR 9.8 yrs with RA	4 weekly (2h) sessions Optional home visit 2 wks post 1 month 4-8 patients + spouses invited	SME	1 leader Rheumatology OT	Usual care

Group Visits Focusing on Education for the Management of Chronic Conditions in Adults

Study	Sample size Setting *Program name, if applicable*	Demographics: Mean age % male % minority Mean disease duration	GV structure: # Visits, frequency Duration Group size	GV content: SME (self-mgmt) DE (didactic) EE (experiential)	GV leaders: Number of leaders Profession type	Comparator(s)
Hammond, 2008[23]	N=167 UK *LMAP*	55.4 yrs 35% Race NR 7.4 yrs with RA	GV1: 9 sessions (2.5h) over 9 mo 12 months 6-10 patients GV2: 5 (2h) sessions 1.25 months 8-12 patients	GV1: SME, EE GV2: DE, EE	3 leaders Rheumatology OT, community OT, rheumatology PT	GV2
Hewlett, 2011[38]	N=127 UK	59.2 yrs 27% Race NR 14 yrs with RA	GV1: 6 weekly (2h) sessions 1 booster session (wk 14) 1.5 months 4-9 patients GV2: 1 (1h) session Delivered by RA nurse	GV1: SME GV2: DE	2 leaders Clinical psychologist, specialist OT	GV2
Kaplan, 1981[39]	N=34 US	48.2 yrs 0% 9% nonwhite Duration NR	GV1: 1 (2.5h) education session 12 weekly (1-2h) counseling 4 months GV2: 1 (2.5h) education session Group size NR	GV1: DE, counseling GV2: DE	2 leaders Patient counselor, psychiatrist	GV2
Lorig, 1985[40]	N=286 US	67.4 yrs 17% 3% nonwhite Duration NR	6 sessions (2h) over 4 months 4 months 15-20 patients + family	SME	2 leaders Trained peer leaders	Usual care
Lorig, 1999[41]	N=331 US *ASMP*	62.5 yrs 16% 100% Latino Duration NR	6 sessions (2h) over 6 weeks 1.5 months 10-15 patients and family	SME	Lay leaders	Usual care
Lorig, 2004[29]	N=341 US *ASMP*	65.2 yrs 25% 10% nonwhite Duration NR	6 weekly (2h) sessions 1.5 months Group size NR	SME	2 leaders Trained peer leaders	*SMART* group: mailed individual self-management program

Group Visits Focusing on Education for the Management of Chronic Conditions in Adults

Study	Sample size Setting *Program name, if applicable*	Demographics: Mean age % male % minority Mean disease duration	GV structure: # Visits, frequency Duration Group size	GV content: SME (self-mgmt) DE (didactic) EE (experiential)	GV leaders: Number of leaders Profession type	Comparator(s)
Riemsma, 2003[42]	N=218 Netherlands	56.4 yrs 38% Race NR 11.7 yrs with RA	5 weekly (2h) sessions 3 (2h) booster sessions 1.25 months 8 patients +/- spouses	GV1: SME, EE (patients only) GV2: SME, EE (spouses included)	2 leaders RA nurse, nurse	GV2, and Usual care+: self-help guide
Sevick, 2009[43] *ADAPT*	N=316 US	69 yrs 28% 24% nonwhite Duration NR	GV1: 3x month, months 1-4 Biweekly, months 5-6 Monthly, months 7-18 18 months GV2: GV1 structure + 3x/week grp exercise, months 1-4 Group sizes NR	GV1: DE GV2: DE, exercise	NR	GV2, and Healthy lifestyle group: Monthly (1h) DE GV, months 1-3; monthly phone contact, months 4-5; bimonthly phone contact months 6-18
Taal, 1993[44]	N=75 Netherlands	49.6 yrs 20% Race NR 4.3 yrs with RA	5 weekly (2h) sessions 1.25 months 6-8 patients	SME, EE	2 leaders RA nurse, physiotherapist, or social worker	Usual care+: individual referral to physiotherapist

History of falls

Study	Sample size Setting *Program name, if applicable*	Demographics: Mean age % male % minority Mean disease duration	GV structure: # Visits, frequency Duration Group size	GV content: SME (self-mgmt) DE (didactic) EE (experiential)	GV leaders: Number of leaders Profession type	Comparator(s)
Arnold, 2010[45]	N=83 Canada	74.5 yrs 29% Race NR 7.6 yrs with hip pain	GV1: 22 semiweekly (1.5h) sessions 2.75 months GV2: 22 semiweekly (.75h) sessions 2.75 months Group sizes NR	GV1: DE, EE, aquatic exercise GV2: EE, aquatic exercise	2 leaders Aquatic fitness instructor, PT	Usual care, and GV2
Clemson, 2004[24] *Stepping On*	N=310 Australia	78.4 yrs 26% Race NR Duration NR	7 (2h) sessions over 7 weeks 1 (1.5h) booster (after 3mo) 1.75 months 12 patients	DE, EE	OT with geriatrics experience, team of content experts for educational areas	Usual care+: ≤2 home social visits from OT student instructed not to discuss falls or falls prevention
Ryan, 1996[46]	N=45 US	78 yrs 0% 66% black Duration NR	1 (1h) session 1 day 7-8 women	DE	1 leader Nurse	Individual visit, and Usual care+: Health promotion session with no falls prevention info
Shumway-Cook, 2007[25]	N=454 US	75.6 yrs 23% 4% nonwhite Duration NR	6 monthly (1h) sessions 6 months Group size NR	DE, exercise	1 leader Nurse	Usual care (two CDC informational brochures)

Group Visits Focusing on Education for the Management of Chronic Conditions in Adults

Table 2. Findings from interventions reporting standardized or validated measures that compare group visits to control, stratified by clinical areas of arthritis or falls

Study	Outcome	Findings by time period*				GV duration	# Sessions	% Participation†/ % Loss to follow-up‡	Study quality
		0-3 mo	4-6 mo	7-12 mo	13+ mo				
Arthritis									
Self-efficacy									
Ackerman, 2012[31]	heiQ	+	NR	≈	NR	1.5 mo	6	25 / 22	Poor
Barlow, 2000[32]	ASES (pain)	NR	+	NR	NR	1.5 mo	6	NR / 22	Fair
Breedland, 2011[33]	ASES	≈	NR	NR	NR	2 mo	24	NR / 6	Good
Buszewicz, 2006[34]	ASES	NR	+	+	NR	1.5 mo	6	30 / 24	Fair
Giraudet Le Quintrec, 2007[37]	AIII (coping)	NR	NR	–	NR	2 mo + booster @ 4 mo	9	18 / 9	Fair
Hammond, 1999[23]	ASES	Unclear	NR	NR	NR	1 mo	4	NR / 31	Fair
Lorig, 1985[40]	Knowledge + self-management scale	NR	+	NR	NR	4 mo	6	NA / 16	Fair
Lorig, 1999[41]	ASES	NR	+	NR	NR	1.5 mo	6	NR / 17	Poor
Riemsma, 2003[42]	ASES	≈	≈	≈	NR	1.25 mo+ booster @ 3, 6, 9 mo	8	26 / 17	Fair
Taal, 1993[44]	ASES (pain, other)	≈	≈	NR	≈	1.25	5	54 / 24	Poor
	ASES (function)	+	≈	NR	+				
Quality of life/functional status									
Ackerman, 2012[31]	AQoL	≈	NR	≈	NR	1.5 mo	6	25 / 22	Fair
Barlow, 2000[32]	HADS (depression)	NR	+	NR	NR	1.5 mo	6	NR / 22	Fair
Breedland, 2011[33]	Dutch AIMS	≈	NR	NR	NR	2 mo	24	NR / 6	Good
Buszewicz, 2006[34]	SF-36	NR	NR	≈	NR	1.5 mo	6	30 / 24	Fair
Giraudet-Le Quintrec, 2007[37]	AIMS2	NR	NR	≈	NR	2 mo + booster @ 4 mo	9	18 / 9	Fair
Hammond, 1999[23]	HAQ (function)	Unclear	NR	NR	NR	1 mo	4	NR / 31	Fair
Lorig, 1985[40]	HAQ (disability)	NR	≈	NR	NR	4 mo	6	NA / 16	Fair
Lorig, 1999[41]	HAQ (disability)	NR	+	NR	NR	1.5 mo	6	NR / 17	Poor
Patel, 2009[35]	SF-36 / QALY	≈	≈	≈	NR	1.5 mo	6	30 / 21	Fair
Riemsma, 2003[42]	Dutch AIMS2	≈	≈	≈	NR	1.25 mo+ booster @ 3, 6, 9 mo	8	26 / 17	Fair
Taal, 1993[44]	Dutch AIMS	≈	?	NR	≈	1.25 mo	5	54 / 24	Poor
Biophysical and performance measures									
Breedland, 2011[33]	VO₂ max	+	NR	NR	NR	2 mo	24	NR / 6	Good
Utilization									
Ackerman, 2012[31]	MD visits	≈	NR	≈	NR	1.5 mo	6	25 / 22	Fair
Barlow, 2000[32]	MD visits	NR	≈	NR	NR	1.5 mo	6	NR / 22	Fair

Group Visits Focusing on Education for the Management of Chronic Conditions in Adults

Study	Outcome	Findings by time period*				GV duration	# Sessions	% Participation†/ % Loss to follow-up‡	Study quality
		0-3 mo	4-6 mo	7-12 mo	13+ mo				
Buszewicz, 2006[34]	MD visits	NR	NR	≈	NR	1.5 mo	6	30 / 24	Fair
Lorig, 1985[40]	MD visits	NR	≈	NR	NR	4 mo	6	NA / 16	Fair
Lorig, 1999[41]	MD visits	NR	+	NR	NR	1.5 mo	6	NR / 17	Poor
Patel, 2009[35]	MD/outpatient visits	NR	≈	≈	NR	1.5 mo	6	30 / 24	Fair
History of falls									
Self-efficacy									
Arnold, 2010[45]	ABC (falls efficacy)	+	NR	NR	NR	2.75 mo	22	55 / 23	Fair
Clemson, 2004[24]	MES	NR	NR	NR	+	1.75 mo + booster @ 3 mo	8	NA / 15	Good
Quality of life/functional status									
Arnold, 2010[45]	AIMS2	≈	NR	NR	NR	2.75 mo	22	55 / 23	Fair
Clemson, 2004[24]	SF-36	NR	NR	NR	≈	1.75 mo + booster @ 3 mo	8	NA / 15	Good
Biophysical and performance measures									
Arnold, 2010[45]	TUG (dual task)	≈	NR	NR	NR	2.75 mo	22	55 / 23	Fair
Clemson, 2004[24]	Fall events	NR	NR	NR	+	1.75 mo + booster @ 3 mo	8	NA / 15	Good
Ryan, 1996[46]	Fall events	Unclear	NR	NR	NR	1 day	1	NR / NR	Poor
Shumway-Cook, 2007[25]	Fall events	NR	NR	≈	NR	6 mo	6	88 / 5	Fair
	TUG	NR	NR	+	NR				

*Symbols pertain to statistical significance (p<0.05), as follows: ≈ denotes no difference between arms; + denotes in favor of the GV arm; - denotes in favor of the C arm; NR = data not reported for time period.
†Defined as percent eligible for enrollment among those invited to participate.
‡Defined as percent lost to follow up among those randomized.

Group Visits Focusing on Education for the Management of Chronic Conditions in Adults

Table 3. Summary of findings from head-to-head group visit interventions and group vs. individual visit interventions for arthritis or falls

Study	Arm 1	Arm 2	% Participation*/ % Loss to follow-up†	Study quality (Good/ Fair/ Poor)	Key findings
Arthritis					
Hewlett, 2011[38]	GV1 (7 SME sessions)	GV2 (1 DE session)	15 / 24	Good	Beneficial effect of cognitive behavior therapy relative to didactic-only single session GV assessed at 4.5 months
Ettinger, 1997[22]	GV1 (3 DE sessions)	GV2 aerobic exercise (36 classes)	53 / 17	Fair	Beneficial effect of either exercise group vs. education group on pain, disability, and functional performance. Dose response for patients who completed more sessions of either exercise program.
	GV1 (3 DE sessions)	GV3 resistance exercise (36 classes)			
Freeman, 2002[36]	GV1 (4 SME sessions)	GV2 (4 DE sessions)	94 / 23	Fair	Cognitive-behavioral education program did not significantly improve pain or self efficacy for patients newly diagnosed with RA.
Hammond, 2008[47]	GV1 (9 SME, EE sessions)	GV2 (5 DE, EE sessions)	46 / 37	Fair	GV1 was effective in improving short-term pain, functional disability, self-efficacy, and reducing physician visits compared to GV2. Longer-term benefits for GV1 for pain, and maintained functional ability compared to declines in GV2.
Kaplan, 1981[39]	GV1 (13 DE, group counseling sessions)	GV2 (1 DE session)	NR / 35	Poor	Combination of education and short-term group counseling led to improved knowledge and self-esteem.
Lorig, 2004[29]	GV (6 SME sessions)	Mailed individual program	84 / 32	Good	Both programs show moderate improvements in self-efficacy, pain, and disability outcomes. Earlier advantages of mailed program narrowed after 3 yrs. GV program had decreased physician visits compared with mailed program.
Riemsma, 2003[42]	GV1 (8 SME, EE sessions) Patients only	GV2 (8 SME, EE sessions) Patients and significant others	26 / 17	Fair	Participation of significant others led to decreases in self-efficacy for coping with other symptoms compared to improvements in patients participating without their partners.
Sevick, 2009[43]	GV1 (28 DE sessions)	GV2 (76 DE, exercise sessions)	NR / 20	Good	GV2 was the most effective in improving function and pain when costs were not considered. GV1 was the most cost-effective for reducing weight; GV2 was the most cost-effective for improving function.
	GV1 (28 DE sessions)	GV3 (3 DE sessions)			
History of falls					
Arnold, 2010[15]	GV1 (22 DE, EE, aquatic exercise classes)	GV2 (22 EE, aquatic exercise classes)	55 / 23	Fair	Combination of aquatic exercise and education resulted in improvements in functional performance vs. aquatic exercise alone.
Ryan, 1996[46]	GV (1 DE)	Individual (1 DE)	NR / NR	Poor	Small study. Control group experienced the most falls in the post period.

*Defined as percent eligible for enrollment among those invited to participate.
†Defined as percent lost to follow-up among those randomized.

Asthma, COPD

Five studies conducted in the US or Australia examined the effects of group visit interventions compared with usual care in patients with asthma (Table 4).[48-52] The group interventions involved didactic education in four studies[49-52] and self-management education in one study.[48] Decreased utilization was observed in two studies,[48,51] and improvements in quality of life measures were noted in two studies.[48,49] The studies were limited by selection bias and other methodological issues, however, and study quality was fair to poor.

Five studies of group visits in COPD patients were conducted in a variety of settings: Northern Ireland,[53] the UK,[54] the Netherlands,[55] France,[56] and a VA Medical Center in the US.[57] Three studies compared didactic education combined with exercise training to DE alone[54,55] or to usual care.[56] Two other studies examined the effects of SME compared with DE,[57] usual care,[53] or individual support.[53] The group education sessions were held weekly or biweekly for four to eight weeks, and two studies with exercise components continued the exercise sessions monthly for up to a year (Table 4).[54,55] Better exercise capacity was observed in the studies that combined exercise training with DE, as compared with usual care[56] or with DE alone (Tables 5 and 6).[54,55] One of these was a small, good-quality study that also found the intervention improved the symptom subscale of the St. George's Respiratory Questionnaire but not activity level.[56] In a smoking cessation intervention study, five weeks of SME group sessions had no effect on smoking cessation at 12 months, compared with usual care.[53] A study comparing DE group visits with cognitive-behavioral therapy SME group visits among US Veterans with COPD found that both types of group visits significantly improved QOL, anxiety, depression, and 6MWD, with no significant differences between groups.[57]

Overall, a small body of fair-to-good quality evidence suggests that group exercise training in combination with didactic education may be associated with small improvements or less decline over time in exercise capacity and COPD symptoms, though the clinical significance of these findings is unclear. There is little methodologically sound evidence examining the impact of group visits in patients with asthma.

Return to Contents

Group Visits Focusing on Education for the Management of Chronic Conditions in Adults

Table 4. Characteristics of group visit interventions focusing on education for the management of asthma or COPD

Study	Sample size Setting Program name, if applicable	Demographics: Mean age % male % minority Mean disease duration	GV structure: # Visits, frequency Duration Group size	GV content: SME (self-mgmt) DE (didactic) EE (experiential)	GV leaders: Number of leaders Profession type	Comparator
Asthma						
Wilson, 1993[48]	N=323 US	NR	4 weekly sessions 1 month 6-8 patients	SME	1 leader Nurse educator	3 comparators: 1) individual education 2) usual care with workbook 3) usual care with no supplemental education
Abdulwadud, 1999[49]	N=125 Australia Australian Asthma Management Program	Mean age 45.6 40% male Race NR Duration NR	3 weekly sessions 3 weeks Up to 13 patients	DE	1 leader Nurse educator	Usual care
Allen, 1995[50]	N=116 Australia	Mean age 40 46% male Race NR Duration NR	4 weekly sessions 4 weeks 10-12 patients	DE	2 leaders Asthma educators	Usual care
Bolton, 1991[51]	N=241 US	Mean age 38 34% male 67% non-white Duration NR	3 sessions Duration NR 6-10 patients	DE	1 leader Nurse educator	Usual care
Snyder, 1987[52]	N=79 US *Wheezers Anonymous*	Mean age 28 45% male Race NR Duration NR	2 sessions, NOS Duration NR 8-12 patients	DE	1 leader Respiratory therapist	Usual care
COPD						
Wilson, 2008[53]	N=91 Northern Ireland	Mean age 61 48% male Race NR Duration NR Current smokers	5 weekly sessions 5 weeks total N per session NR	SME	1 leader Respiratory Nurse Specialist	Usual care (n=35), Individual support (n=27)

Group Visits Focusing on Education for the Management of Chronic Conditions in Adults

Study	Sample size Setting *Program name, if applicable*	Demographics: Mean age % male % minority Mean disease duration	GV structure: # Visits, frequency Duration Group size	GV content: SME (self-mgmt) DE (didactic) EE (experiential)	GV leaders: Number of leaders Profession type	Comparator
Kunik, 2008[57]	N=238 US VAMC	Mean age 66 96% male 16% Black 3% Hispanic	8 weekly sessions 8 weeks Up to 10 patients	SME: CBT	1 leader Psychology intern or post-doctoral fellow with CBT experience	DE group education
Bestall, 2003[54]	N=66 UK	Mean age 69 51% male Race NR Duration NR	16 DE bi-weekly sessions, 8 weeks total (both groups), followed by 10 EE monthly sessions, 1 year total (exercise group only) N per session NR	DE + EE: exercise	NR	DE group education
Effing, 2011[55]	N=159 Netherlands *COPE-active*	Mean age 63 58% male Race NR Duration NR 35% smokers	DE: 4 weekly sessions/1 month total; 5 patients EE: 2-3 times/week, 11 months total; 2-3 patients	DE + EE: exercise	2 leaders Respiratory nurse Physiotherapist	DE group education
Ninot, 2011[56]	N=45 France	Mean age 63 84% male Race NR Duration NR 26% smokers	8 sessions, 2x week 4 weeks total	DE + EE: exercise	2 leaders DE led by health professional, EE led by exercise trainer	Usual care

Group Visits Focusing on Education for the Management of Chronic Conditions in Adults

Table 5. Findings from interventions comparing group visits to usual care control for the management of Asthma or COPD, stratified by clinical area and outcome category

Study	Outcome	Findings by time period*				GV duration	#visits	% Participation†/ % Loss to follow-up‡	Study quality
		0-3 mo	4-6 mo	7-12 mo	13+ mo				
Asthma									
Self-efficacy									
Abdulwadud, 1999[49]	Asthma Attitudes and Beliefs Questionnaire	NR	≈	NR	NR	3 weeks	3	71 / 38	Poor
Quality of life/functional status									
Abdulwadud, 1999[49]	AQLQ	+	≈	NR	NR	3 weeks	3	71 / 38	Poor
Wilson, 1993[48]	Asthma bother scale	NR	NR	+	NR	3-4 months	4	56 / 14	Fair
Utilization									
Wilson, 1993[48]	Acute visits	NR	NR	≈	+	1 month	4	56 / 14	Fair
Bolton, 1991[51]	ER visits	NR	+	≈	NR	NR	3	45 / 7	Fair
COPD									
Quality of life/functional status									
Wilson, 2008[53]	Smoking cessation	NR	NR	≈	NR	5 weeks	5	60 / NR	Fair
Ninot, 2011[56]	SGRQ	NR	NR	≈§	NR	4 weeks	8	NA / 16	Good
Biophysical and performance measures									
Kunik, 2008[57]	6MWD	≈	NR	≈	NR	8 weeks	8	19 / 55	Good
Ninot, 2011[56]	6MWD	NR	NR	+	NR	4 weeks	8	NA / 16	Good
Utilization									
Ninot, 2011[56]	Days in hospital for COPD admission	NR	NR	≈	NR	4 weeks	8	NA / 16	Good

*Symbols pertain to statistical significance (p<0.05), as follows: ~ denotes no difference between arms, ↓ denotes in favor of the GV arm; - denotes in favor of the C arm; NR = data not reported for time period.
†Defined as percent eligible for enrollment among those invited to participate.
‡Defined as percent lost to follow up among those randomized.
§There was a greater decrease in total SGRQ score in GV compared with usual control, but the difference did not reach statistical significance (p=0.06). There was a significantly greater reduction on the SGRQ Symptom subscale associated with GV, but no significant differences in the Activity or Impacts subscales.

Group Visits Focusing on Education for the Management of Chronic Conditions in Adults

Table 6. Summary of findings from head-to-head group visit interventions and group vs. individual visit interventions for the management of asthma or COPD

Study	Arm 1	Arm 2	% Participation†/ % Loss to follow-up‡	Study quality (Good/ Fair/ Poor)	Key findings
Asthma					
Wilson, 1993[48]	GV (3 SME sessions)	IV (3-5 weekly SME sessions)	56 / 14	Fair	No significant differences between GV and IV. GV and IV were equally effective compared with UC. Reduced bother and improved MDI technique observed with both small group and individual education.
COPD					
Bestall 2003[54]	GV (16 DE + 26 EE sessions: exercise)	GV (16 DE sessions)	NR / 16	Fair	Compared with DE alone, pts in exercise group had improved exercise capacity (shuttle walking distance) that lasted 6 months. For QoL (CRQ, SGRQ) there were mixed results at 6 months, and no differences between groups at 1 year.
Effing 2011[55]	GV (4 DE + up to 120 EE sessions)	GV (4 DE sessions)	41 / 11	Fair	COPE-active group experienced an improvement in maximal exercise capacity compared to the steady decline in the control group.
Kunik, 2008[57]	GV (8 DE sessions)	GV (8 SME sessions: CBT)	19 / 55	Good	CBT and COPD education groups were comparable and significantly improved QoL, anxiety, depression, and 6MWD, with no significant differences between groups, and improvement was maintained till the end of the study (52 weeks).

Hypertension, CHF, CAD

Our literature search identified two fair-quality studies of group visit interventions conducted in patients with CHF or CAD,[58,59] and one good-quality study published in two reports[27,60] (Table 7). One study compared cardiac education lectures with usual care in US Veterans with moderately severe CHF, and found no difference in quality of life after 15 weeks of DE sessions.[59] A study conducted in a non-Veteran US population used cognitive-behavioral change counseling to increase exercise maintenance in patients with MI, CABG or angioplasty, and found that subjects in the usual care group were significantly more likely to stop exercising in the year following completion of a cardiac rehabilitation program compared with subjects in the intervention group, although standardized self-efficacy measures indicated no differences between groups (Table 8).[58] The study conducted in the Netherlands[27,60] used the Chronic Disease Self-Management Program (CDSMP) developed by Lorig and colleagues for the management of multiple chronic diseases.[61] The CDSMP was associated with short-term improvements in cognitive symptom management, self-care behavior, and cardiac-specific QOL among patients with CHF in the Netherlands, but no long-term effects were found.[27,60]

Seven studies examined the effects of group visits on blood pressure in patients with hypertension.[26,62-67] The studies were conducted in a range of international settings, and study quality varied widely (Table 7). Three studies used SME techniques[26,63,66] and three studies used DE[62-64,67] in comparison with usual care or an informational control. One trial compared SME directly with DE.[65] Reductions in blood pressure measurements were noted in all three SME studies[26,63,66] and in one DE study.[62] In the trial comparing SME directly with DE, there were no significant reductions in SBP or DBP found in either group at three months. However, significantly more SME patients had controlled BP, defined as the proportion of patients with mean 24-h BP <140/90 mm Hg, compared with DE (70% vs 44%, p=0.04).

Overall, there were very few studies of group visits in CHF patients, and their findings on self-efficacy, quality of life, and biophysical measures were largely neutral. Group self-management education interventions in patients with hypertension have reported improvements in blood pressure control in short-term and long-term studies, but the overall strength of evidence is low.

Return to Contents

Group Visits Focusing on Education for the Management of Chronic Conditions in Adults

Table 7. Characteristics of group visit interventions focusing on education for the management of congestive heart failure, coronary artery disease, or hypertension

Study	Sample size Setting Program name, if applicable	Demographics: Mean age % male % minority Mean disease duration	GV structure: # Visits, frequency Duration Group size	GV content: SME (self-mgmt) DE (didactic) EE (experiential)	GV leaders: Number of leaders Profession type	Comparator
CHF/CAD						
Smeulders, 2010[27,60]	N=317 Netherlands CDSMP	Mean age 67 73% male Race NR Duration NR	6 weekly sessions 6 weeks total 6-12 patients	SME	2 leaders Cardiac nurse specialist CHF patient peer leader	Usual care
Chang, 2005[59]	N=62 US VAMC	Mean age 69 % male NR 17% non-white Duration NR	15 weekly sessions 15 weeks total Group size NR	DE	Experts on medical, pharmaceutical, lifestyle, nutrition, and psychosocial issues	Usual care
Moore, 2006[58]	N=250 US CHANGE	Mean age 62 17% black 2% non-white, NOS Duration NR	5 sessions: 3 weekly followed by 2 monthly 3 months total 6-8 patients	SME	1 leader Cardiac nurse	Usual care
Hypertension						
Baghianimoghadam, 2010[67]	N=150 Iran	Mean age 57.9 39% male Race NR Duration 6.77 yr	Frequency NR 2 months total Group size NR	DE + EE	1 leader Health education researcher	Usual care
Nessman, 1980[62]	N=52 US VAMC	Mean age 55 10% black 16% Mexican-American Duration NR	8 weekly sessions 8 weeks total Group size NR	DE	2 leaders Nurse, psychologist	Informational control (audiotape)
Rujiwatthanakorn, 2011[63]	N=96 Thailand	Mean age 61 40% male Race NR Duration NR	3 sessions 8 weeks total 6-7 patients Duration NR	SME	1 leader Nurse	Usual care
Balcazar, 2009[64]	N=98 US	Mean age 53 21% male 100% Mexican-American, 87% born in Mexico Duration NR	4 sessions at weeks 1, 2, 3, 8 8 weeks total 15-20 patients	DE	2 leaders Promotoras (Mexican-American community health workers)	Informational control

Group Visits Focusing on Education for the Management of Chronic Conditions in Adults

Study	Sample size Setting *Program name, if applicable*	Demographics: Mean age % male % minority Mean disease duration	GV structure: # Visits, frequency Duration Group size	GV content: SME (self-mgmt) DE (didactic) EE (experiential)	GV leaders: Number of leaders Profession type	Comparator
Figar, 2006[65]	N=60 Argentina *PEM*	Mean age 69 57% male Duration NR	4 weekly sessions 4 weeks 10 patients	SME	Physicians with experience in HTN education/management	DE
Scala, 2008[66]	N=292 Italy	Mean age 62 42% male Race NR Duration NR	3 sessions 4 months total 4-5 patients	SME	1 leader Moderator, tutor assistants	Informational control
Svetkey, 2009[26]	N=574 US	Mean age 60.5 39% male 37% black 1% Hispanic Duration NR	20 weekly sessions 6 months total 10-15 patients	SME	2 leaders Behavioral interventionist, assistants (community health advisors)	Usual care

Table 8. Findings from interventions comparing group visits to usual care control for the management of CHF/CHD/Hypertension, stratified by clinical area and outcome category

Study	Outcome	Findings by time period*				GV duration	Visits	% Participation† / % Loss to follow-up‡	Study quality
		0-3 mo	4-6 mo	7-12 mo	13+ mo				
CHF/CAD									
Self-efficacy									
Smeulders, 2010[27,60]	GSES	≈	≈	≈	NR	6 weeks	6	44 / 16	Good
	Cardiac self-efficacy: KCCQ	≈	≈	≈	NR				
	Cognitive Symptom Scale	+	≈	≈	NR				
Moore, 2006[58]	Index of Self-Regulation; Exercise Barriers and Adherence Self-Efficacy Scale	≈	NR	NR	≈	3 months	5	50 / 19	Fair
Quality of life/functional status									
Smeulders, 2010[27,60]	Cardiac-specific QOL	+	≈	≈	NR	6 weeks	6	44 / 16	Good
	HADS - Anxiety	≈	≈	≈	NR				
	HADS - Depression	≈	≈	≈	NR				
Chang, 2005[59]	Minnesota Living with Heart Failure Questionnaire	NR	≈	NR	NR	15 weeks	15	17 / 13	Fair
Biophysical									
Smeulders, 2010[27,60]	Biophysical: BMI	≈	≈	NR	NR	6 weeks	6	44 / 16	Good
Hypertension									
Biophysical									
Nessman, 1980[62]	SBP and DBP	+	+	NR	NR	8 weeks	4	36 / 0	Poor
Rujiwatthanakorn, 2011[63]	SBP and DBP	+	NR	NR	NR	8 weeks	3	70 / 12	Poor
Balcazar, 2009[64]	BP, BMI & Waist circumference	≈	NR	NR	NR	8 weeks	4	NR / 0	Poor
Scala, 2008[66]	SBP and DBP	NR	NR	NR	+	4 months	3	NR / 42	Poor
Svetkey, 2009[26]	SBP and DBP	NR	+	NR	≈	6 months	20	56 / 12	Good

Table 9. Summary of findings from head-to-head group visit interventions and group vs. individual visit interventions for the management of hypertension

Study	Arm 1	Arm 2	% Participation / % Attrition	Study quality	Key findings
Figar, 2006[65]	GV (4 SME sessions)	GV (4 DE sessions)	NR / 17	Good	More SME patients had controlled BP (defined as the proportion of patients with mean 24-h BP <140/90 mm Hg) compared with DE: 70% vs 44%, p=0.04. No significant reductions in SBP or DBP in either group.

Diabetes Mellitus

We included 30 publications of 29 studies of group visit interventions in patients with DM (Table 10). We conducted meta-analyses of the 17 studies comparing the effects of a group visit intervention to usual care on HbA1c (Figures 3-6). Overall, in 14 studies, group visit interventions reduced HbA1c slightly more over six months of follow-up than usual care, though there was significant heterogeneity which should temper confidence in these results (Figure 3, mean difference HbA1c -0.27%; 95% CI -0.44 to -0.11; I^2=67.1%). At least part of the heterogeneity seemed to be associated with study quality. The two good quality studies found no short-term improvements in HbA1c (mean difference HbA1c 0.02; 95% CI -0.14 to 0.17; I^2=0.0%). Group visit interventions lasting more than three months appeared to have a more pronounced effect on HbA1c improvement than those of shorter duration (-0.49% vs -0.20%), but the quality of these longer duration intervention studies was also lower (Figure 4). We found similar effects on HbA1c at 7 to 12 months in the 10 studies with longer-term follow-up (Figures 5 and 6). Funnel plot analyses showed no evidence of publication bias for 6 month outcomes (Egger bias coefficient=-1.62, 95% CI [-3.73 to 0.48]), but some evidence of publication bias for 12 month outcomes (Egger bias coefficient=-2.14, 95% CI [-3.62 to -0.66]). Multivariate meta-regression models showed that none of the covariates examined—duration of the group visit intervention, study quality, or year of publication—were independently associated with changes in HbA1c.

Five studies found improvements in self-efficacy or illness belief scores with four of these studies finding positive effects beyond six months of follow-up (Table 11). Perhaps not surprisingly, four of the five studies finding beneficial effects on self-efficacy involved interventions specifically focused on broader self-management skills training rather than didactic education.[19,30,68,69]

Despite finding that some interventions may improve self-efficacy, there was little evidence that group visit interventions improved quality of life over the short- or long-term (Table 11). One large, good-quality cluster-randomized trial in patients with newly diagnosed diabetes compared a six-hour self-management skills program to a control group which received equal contact time but no self-management training. Though the intervention was associated with sustained improvements in illness beliefs, there was no detectable effect on quality of life, depression or biomedical outcomes over the long-term.[68,70] Few studies reported or were powered to evaluate utilization outcomes.

Eleven studies compared a group visit intervention to one or more active interventions (Table 12). Three of these studies found that interventions focused on self-management skills training were associated with greater improvements in glycemic control than didactic educational approaches, though there were multiple other differences in the interventions being compared making it difficult to draw firm conclusions about the effects of educational approach alone.[14,71,72] Two studies compared group to individual education: one was a small good-quality trial which found individual education was associated with better outcomes,[73] while the other was a poor-quality study showing similar effects of group and individual education.[74] One fair-quality study found that an automated telephone-based self-management intervention performed similarly to an in-person group self-management skills intervention.[30]

Overall, we found group visit interventions in patients with diabetes may have modest effects on glycemic control over the short- and long-term, but the strength of evidence supporting this conclusion is low mostly because of inconsistencies across studies and methodological weaknesses of the studies finding the most positive effects. Interventions focused on self-management skills training were associated with improved self-efficacy and illness belief scores over the short- and long-term. However, there was no consistent evidence that group visit interventions improved quality of life.

Group Visits Focusing on Education for the Management of Chronic Conditions in Adults

Table 10. Characteristics of group visit interventions focusing on education for the management of diabetes mellitus

Study	Population: Setting Program name, if applicable	Demographics: Mean age % male % minority Mean disease duration	GV structure: # Visits, frequency Duration Group size	GV content: SME (self-mgmt) DE (didactic) EE (experiential)	GV leaders: Number of leaders Profession type	Comparator
Adolfsson, 2007[75]	N=101 Sweden	63.1 yrs 54% Minority NR 6.6 yrs with DM	4 (2.5h) sessions 1 booster (2.5h) within 7 months 5-8 patients	DE	7 physicians and 12 diabetes specialist nurses	Usual care
Anderson, 2005[76]	N=239 US	61 yrs 18% 96% minority 8.5 yrs with DM	6 weekly (2h) sessions 1.5 months Group size NR	SME	Certified diabetes educators	Usual care
Brown, 2002[15]	N=256 US *The Starr County Border Health Initiative*	54 yrs 36 % Race NR 7.85 yrs with DM	12 weekly, 12 biweekly, 3 monthly (2h) sessions 12 months Group size NR	DE, EE	Bilingual Mexican American nurses, dietitians, local community workers	Usual care
Brown, 2005[16]*	N=216 US *The Starr County Border Health Initiative*	49.6 yrs 40% Race NR 5.1 yrs with DM	GV1: 3 weekly, 12 biweekly, 3 monthly (2h) sessions 12 months Group size NR GV2: 8 weekly (2h) sessions 3 support @ 3, 6, and 12 months 8 patients	DE, EE	Bilingual Mexican American nurses, dietitians, local community workers	GV2
De Greef, 2011[73]	N=67 Belgium	67.4 yrs 70.1% Minority NR 64.5% diagnosed <5 yr	3 (1.5h) sessions every 3wks 3 months Group size NR	SME	Clinical psychologist	Usual care; individual visit arm: 3 (15min) visits with similar content to GV

Group Visits Focusing on Education for the Management of Chronic Conditions in Adults

Evidence-based Synthesis Program

Study	Population: Setting *Program name, if applicable*	Demographics: Mean age % male % minority Mean disease duration	GV structure: # Visits, frequency Duration Group size	GV content: SME (self-mgmt) DE (didactic) EE (experiential)	GV leaders: Number of leaders Profession type	Comparator
Deakin, 2006[71]*	N=314 UK	61.6 yrs Gender NR Race NR 6.7 yrs with DM	6 weekly (2h) sessions 1.5 months 16 patients (mean)	SME	1 diabetes research dietitian/ educator	Usual care+: diabetes education and review with individual appointments with a dietitian (30 min), practice nurse (15 min) and physician (10 min)
Dejesus, 2009[77]*	N=54 US	76% aged 60+ 48% Race NR Duration NR	1 session 7 patients	DE	Diabetes nurse educator	Usual care
Hornsten, 2008[17]	N=104 Sweden	63 yrs 54% Race NR All diagnosed ≤ 2yrs	10 (2h) sessions over 9 mo 9 months 5-8 patients	SME	Diabetes nurses	Usual care
Khunti, 2012[68] Davies, 2008[70]	N=824 UK *DESMOND*	59.5 yrs 55% male 6% minority Duration NR	1 (6h) session 1 day or 2 half-days Group size NR	SME	Healthcare professional	Usual care+: (resources to provide equivalent contact time as intervention)
Kulzer, 2007[72]*	N=193 Germany	Mean age 55.6 50.3% male Race NR Mean duration 6.6 yrs	GV1: 4 DE sessions GV2: 12 SME sessions GV3: 6 SME sessions + 6 IV Duration NR Group size 6-10	GV1: DE GV2: SME	Health psychologist	Self-management education - 6 90 min group lessons and 6 90 min individual lessons
Lorig, 2009[69]	N=345 US *DSMP*	66.55 yrs 35.7% 32.7% minority Duration NR	6 weekly (2.5h) sessions 1.5 months 10-15 patients	SME	Peer leaders	Usual care
Lujan, 2007[78]	N=150 US	58 yrs 20% 100% Mexican origin Duration NR	8 weekly (2h) sessions 2 months 6 patients (English class) 23 patients (Spanish class)	DE	2 leaders Promotoras, nurses, dietitians, social workers	Usual care (2 pamphlets)

Group Visits Focusing on Education for the Management of Chronic Conditions in Adults

Evidence-based Synthesis Program

Study	Population: Setting *Program name, if applicable*	Demographics: Mean age % male % minority *Mean disease duration*	GV structure: # Visits, frequency Duration Group size	GV content: SME (self-mgmt) DE (didactic) EE (experiential)	GV leaders: Number of leaders Profession type	Comparator
Melkus, 2010[13]*	N=109 UK	46 yrs 0% 100% minority Duration NR	11 weekly (1-2h) sessions 3 months Group size NR	SME	Nurse practitioner	Culturally neutral group DE (10 weekly sessions)
Miller, 2002[79]	N=98 US	72.5 yrs 47% 17% black 7.2 yrs	GV1: 10 weekly (1.5-2h) sessions 2.5 months Group size NR GV2: Offered 6 (2h) sessions Group size NR	GV1: DE, EE GV2: DE	Dietitian	GV2 (participants were mailed printed material if they did not attend the group session)
Philis-Tsimikas, 2011[18]	N=207 US *Project Dulce*	50.7 years 29% male Minority NR Duration NR	8 weekly (2h) sessions 8 monthly support groups 10 months Group size NR	DE	Trained peer educator	Usual care
Raji, 2002[80]*	N=106 US VAMC	Mean age 60 yrs 99% male Race NR Duration NR	4 daily sessions 4 sequential days 4-6 patients	DE	Physician, nurse, nutritionist, pharmacist, exercise physiologist, social worker, and diabetes educator	2 comparators: passive education and no-intervention
Rickheim, 2002[74]*	N=170 US	Mean age 52.5 34% male Race 7% non-white? Duration 0.9 yrs	4 sessions (at 0, 2 wks, 3 mo, 6 mo) 6 months total	DE	A diabetes nurse specialist (RN) and diabetes nutrition specialist (RD)	Individual education sessions
Rosal, 2011[19]	N=252 US *Latinos en Control*	83.7% aged 45+ 23.4% 87.7% minority 31.3% diagnosed <5 yr	12 weekly + 8 monthly First session (1h) individual Remaining (2.5h) group 11 months Group size NR	SME, EE	Nutritionist or health educator and lay leader or 3 supervised lay leaders	Usual care
Rygg, 2012[21]	N=146 Norway	66 yrs 55% 0% 5 yrs with DM	3 biweekly (5h) sessions 1.25 months 8-10 patients	DE, EE	Diabetes nurses; also included physician, physiotherapist, nutritionist, and lay person	Usual care

Group Visits Focusing on Education for the Management of Chronic Conditions in Adults

Study	Population: Setting *Program name, if applicable*	Demographics: Mean age % male % minority Mean disease duration	GV structure: # Visits, frequency Duration Group size	GV content: SME (self-mgmt) DE (didactic) EE (experiential)	GV leaders: Number of leaders Profession type	Comparator
Sarkadi, 2004[81]*	N=77 Sweden	Mean age 66 % male NR Race NR Duration 5.9 yrs treatment; 2.6 yrs control	12 monthly sessions 1 year total Group size NR	DE	Pharmacists trained to be facilitators, and a nurse specialist	Usual care
Scain, 2009[82]	N=104 Brazil	59 yrs 47% 9.4% black 10.5 yrs	4 weekly (2h) sessions 1 month 8-10 patients	DE	NR	Usual care
Schillinger, 2009[30]	N=339 US *IDEALL*	56.1 years 41% male 92.3% minority Duration NR	9 monthly (1.5h) sessions 9 months 6-10 patients	SME	2 leaders Physician and language-concordant health educator	Usual care; automated telephone self-management support group (39 weekly, automated calls over 9 months, nurse phone follow-up)
Sharifirad, 2012[83]	N=97 Iran *BASNEF*	67.05 yrs 35% Minority NR 14 yrs with DM	4 (70min) sessions 1 month Group size NR	DE	Physician, specialist of endocrine disorder, diabetes nurse, and nutritionist	Usual care
Sperl-Hillen, 2011[84]*	N=623 US *IDEA*	Mean age 61.8 50.6% male 22.1% Hispanic 5.5% Black Duration 11.7 yrs	4 weekly sessions 4 weeks total 1-10 patients (mean 5)	DE	Nurses and dietitians trained to facilitate GE sessions	3 individual education sessions at 1-month intervals
Steed, 2005[85]	N=127 UK *UCL-DSMP*	59.8 yrs 71.2% male 51% minority 10.8 years	5 weekly (2.5h) sessions 1 booster (2.5h) @ 3 months 1.25 months Group size NR	SME	Diabetes specialist nurses and dietitians	Usual care
Surwit, 2002[20]*	N=108 US	Mean age 57.4 58.3% male 8.3% Black 1% Asian	5 weekly sessions 5 weeks total Group size NR	EE	NR	DE group visits

Group Visits Focusing on Education for the Management of Chronic Conditions in Adults

Study	Population: Setting *Program name, if applicable*	Demographics: Mean age % male % minority Mean disease duration	GV structure: # Visits, frequency Duration Group size	GV content: SME (self-mgmt) DE (didactic) EE (experiential)	GV leaders: Number of leaders Profession type	Comparator
Toobert, 2011[86,87]	N=280 US ¡Viva Bien!	57.11 yrs 0% 100% minority 10.4 yrs with DM	2.5-day retreat + 36 weekly and biweekly sessions 12 months Group size NR	DE, EE	Bilingual physician, dietitian, exercise instructor, bilingual facilitator	Usual care
Weinger, 2011[114]*	N=222 US	52.5 yrs 49.5% 10.3% minority 17.2 yrs with DM	5 (2h) sessions over 6 wks 1.5 months Group size NR	SME	Certified diabetes educator	Unlimited access to individual DM nurse and dietitian visits
Zapotoczky, 2001[88]*	N=34 Austria	Mean age 62 yrs 36% male	12 monthly sessions 1 year total 18 patients	DE	Clinical dietitian	All subjects received 4-wk group education. Controls received usual care with no further group education.

* Not included in meta-analysis.

Group Visits Focusing on Education for the Management of Chronic Conditions in Adults

Table 11. Findings from interventions reporting standardized or validated measures that compare group visits to usual care in the management of diabetes mellitus

Study	Outcome	Findings by time period*				GV duration	# Sessions	% Participation†/ % Loss to follow-up‡	Study quality (Good/ Fair/ Poor)
		0-3 mo	4-6 mo	7-12 mo	13+ mo				
Self-efficacy									
Brown, 2002[15]	Study specific health belief scale (control)	≈	NR	≈	NR	12 months	27	NR / NR	Poor
Adolfsson, 2007[75]	Study specific questionnaire	NR	NR	≈	NR	7 months (max)	5	53 / 13	Fair
Khunti, 2012[68] Davies, 2008[70]	IPQ-R	+	+	+	+	1 day or 2 half-days	1	NA / 11	Good
Lorig, 2009[69]	PAM	NR	+	NR	NR	1.5 months	6	NA / 15	Fair
	Diabetes Self-Efficacy scale	NR	+	NR	NR				
Lujan, 2007[78]	DHBM	≈	+§	NR	NR	2 months	8	NR / 6	Fair
Rosal, 2011[19]	Study specific scale (diet & physical activity change)	NR	+	+	NR	11 months	19	57 / 16	Fair
Rygg, 2012[21]	PAM	NR	≈	≈	NR	1.25 months	3	91 / 9	Fair
Schillinger, 2009[30]	DQIP	NR	NR	+	NR	9 months	9	73 / 10	Fair
Steed, 2005[85]	MDS (total)	≈	NR	NR	NR	1.25 months + booster @ 3 months	6	51 / 16	Poor
Toobert, 2011[86]	COCSC	NR	+	+	NR	12 months	37	61 / 22	Fair
Quality of life/functional status									
Adolfsson, 2007[75]	Adapted WHO QOL	NR	NR	≈	NR	7 months (max)	5	53 / 13	Fair
Khunti, 2012[68] Davies, 2008[70]	WHO QOL-BREF	NR	NR	NR	≈	1 day or 2 half-days	1	NA / 11	Good
	HADS	≈	≈	+	≈				
Lorig, 2009[69]	PHQ-9 (depression)	NR	+	NR	NR	1.5 months	6	NA / 15	Fair
Rygg, 2012[21]	SF-36 (physical)	NR	≈	≈	NR	1.25 months	3	91 / 9	Fair
	SF-36 (mental)	NR	≈	≈	NR				
	EQ-5D	NR	≈	≈	NR				
Schillinger, 2009[30]	SF-12 (physical)	NR	NR	≈	NR	9 months	9	73 / 10	Fair
	SF-12 (mental)	NR	NR	≈	NR				
Steed, 2005[85]	ADDQOL	+	NR	NR	NR	1.25 months + booster @ 3 months	6	51 / 16	Poor
	SF-36	≈	NR	NR	NR				
Toobert, 2011[86]	CDC Healthy Days (physical)	NR	≈	≈	NR	12 months	37	61 / 22	Fair
	CDC Healthy Days (mental)	NR	≈	≈	NR				

Group Visits Focusing on Education for the Management of Chronic Conditions in Adults

Evidence-based Synthesis Program

Study	Outcome	Findings by time period*				GV duration	# Sessions	% Participation†/ % Loss to follow-up‡	Study quality (Good/ Fair/ Poor)
		0-3 mo	4-6 mo	7-12 mo	13+ mo				
Biophysical and performance measures ǁ									
Dejesus, 2009[77]	Systolic blood pressure	NR	≈	NR	NR	1 day	1	13 / 55	Poor
Utilization									
Dejesus, 2009[77]	RN and MD visits	NR	≈	NR	NR	1 day	1	13 / 55	Poor
Lorig, 2009[69]	MD visits	NR	≈	NR	NR	1.5 months	6	NA / 15	Fair
	ED visits	NR	≈	NR	NR				
	Days hospitalized	NR	≈	NR	NR				
Rygg, 2012[21]	Clinician visits	NR	≈	≈	NR	1.25 months	3	91 / 9	Fair

*Symbols pertain to statistical significance p<0.05: ≈ indicates no difference between arms; + indicates in favor of the GV arm; - indicates in favor of the C arm; NR = not reported.
†Defined as percent eligible for enrollment among those invited to participate.
‡Defined as percent lost to follow-up among those randomized.
§Both groups experienced poorer outcome change with the intervention group experiencing less of a decline.
ǁFive of the seventeen studies included for meta-analysis of mean change in HbA1c did not report quality of life, self-efficacy, or utilization outcomes.[17,18,79,82,83] As a result, these studies are not represented in Table 11.

Return to Contents

Group Visits Focusing on Education for the Management of Chronic Conditions in Adults

Table 12. Summary of findings from head-to-head group visit interventions and group vs. individual visit interventions for the management of diabetes mellitus

Study	Arm 1	Arm 2	% Participation¹/ % Loss to follow-up²	Study quality (Good/Fair/Poor)	Key findings
Deakin, 2006[71]	GV (6 SME)	Individual (3 DE)	20 / 32	Fair	Significant improvements with group compared with individual visits in glycemic control, total cholesterol level, body weight, BMI and waist circumference, reduced requirement for diabetes medication, increased consumption of fruit and vegetables, enjoyment of food, knowledge of diabetes, self-empowerment, self-management skills and treatment satisfaction.
De Greef, 2011[73]	GV (3 SME)	Individual (3 SME)	78 / 5	Good	No improvement in biophysical health outcomes for patients in the GV arm compared to individual visit arm. Individual visit participants showed significant improvements in waist circumference, FBG, HbA1c, and total cholesterol compared to control arm.
Kulzer, 2007[72]	GV1 (4 DE)	GV2 (12 SME) GV3 (6 Group + 6 individual SME)	50 / 6	Fair	GV2 (SME) had significantly lower HbA1c at 15 months compared with both GV1 (DE) and GV3 (group + individual SME). GV2 (SME) also had significant improvements in BMI, anxiety, and exercise relative to GV1 (DE).
Melkus, 2010[13]	GV1 (11 culturally relevant SME)	GV2 (10 culturally neutral DE)	NA / 11	Fair	Both arms had significant, similar reductions in HbA1c at 24 months. The culturally relevant SME group had significantly lower levels of diabetes-related emotional distress at 24 months compared with the culturally neutral DE group.
Miller, 2002[79]	GV1 (10 DE, EE)	GV2 (6 DE, or mailed materials)	NA / 6	Fair	Intense nutrition education GV improved glycemic control
Rickheim, 2002[74]	GV (4 DE)	Individual (4 DE)	NR / 46	Poor	Individual and group education resulted in similar improvements at 6 months in HbA1c, weight, BMI, health-related QOL, attitudes, and medication regimen.
Schillinger, 2009[30]	GV (9 SME)	ATSM: automated telephone self-management (39 SME calls)	73 / 10	Fair	No statistical differences between GV and ATSM arms in self-efficacy, or quality of life (physical). Improvement for ATSM relative to GV in quality of life (mental).
Sperl-Hillen, 2011[84]	GV (4 DE)	Individual (3 DE); Usual care	82 / 2	Fair	HbA1c deceased significantly more with individual DE compared with group DE and usual care. Individual DE significantly reduced distress (PAID) and increased self-efficacy compared with group DE.

Group Visits Focusing on Education for the Management of Chronic Conditions in Adults

Study	Arm 1	Arm 2	% Participation[1]/ % Loss to follow-up[2]	Study quality (Good/ Fair/ Poor)	Key findings
Survit, 2002[20]	GV1 (5 DE)	GV2 (5 DE + EE)	NA / 24	Poor	At 1-year follow-up, patients who received training in stress management in addition to DE had a 0.5% reduction in HbA1c relative to DE alone. No differences between groups in anxiety (STAI) or psychological distress (GHQ; PSS) measures.
Weinger, 2011[14]	GV (5 SME)	Individual DE (unlimited access to DM nurse and dietitian visits)	89 / 3	Fair	GV (SME) had significantly greater reduction in HbA1c levels over 1 year compared with individual DE. No differences in QOL, and self-efficacy measures.
Zapotoczky, 2001[88]	GV1 (4wk + 12mo DE)	GV2 (4wk DE)	100 / 0	Poor	All subjects received 4 wk group education. GV2 received usual care with no further group education. Significant reductions in HbA1c and body weight over 1 year in GV1 (12-month continuation DE) compared with GV2.

[1]% participation from consented=#eligible/#invited
[2]% lost to follow-up of those randomized

Return to Contents

Figure 3. Effect of group visits compared to usual care on HbA1C at ≤6 month follow-up, by study quality

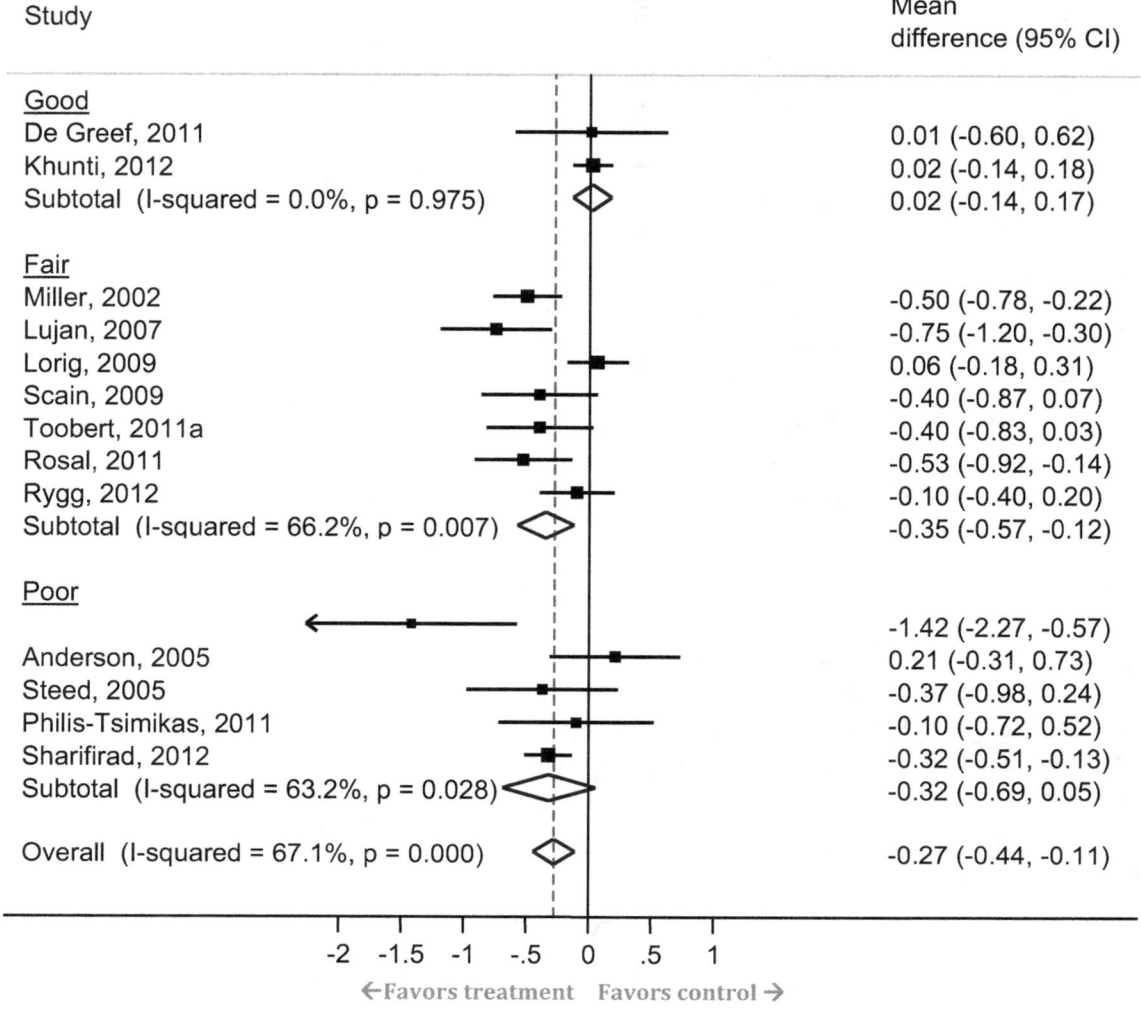

Figure 4. Effect of group visits on HbA1C compared to usual care at ≤6 month follow-up, by duration of intervention

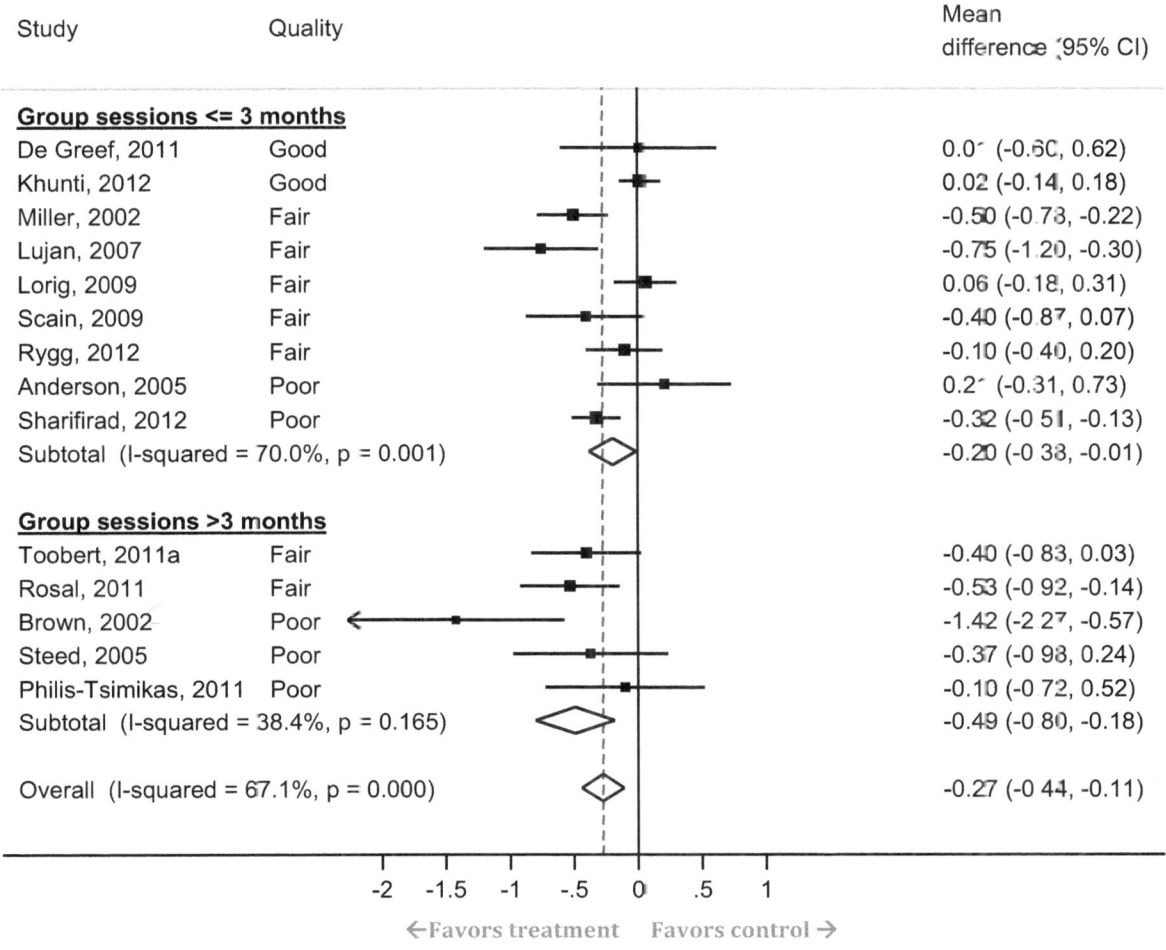

Figure 5. Effect of group visits compared to usual care on HbA1C at 7-12 month follow-up, by study quality

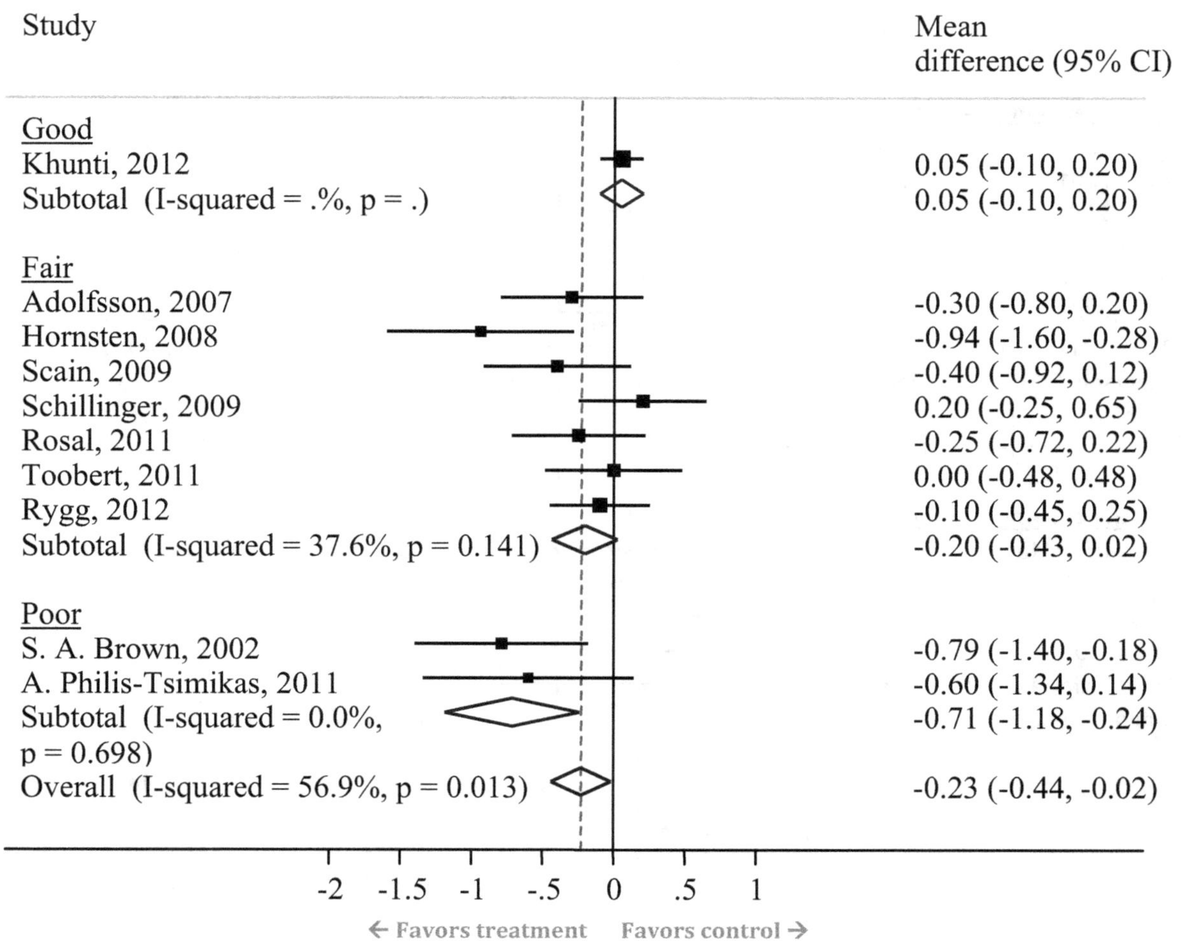

Study
Mean difference (95% CI)
Good
Khunti, 2012
0.05 (-0.10, 0.20)
Subtotal (I-squared = .%, p = .)
0.05 (-0.10, 0.20)
Fair
Adolfsson, 2007
-0.30 (-0.80, 0.20)
Hornsten, 2008
-0.94 (-1.60, -0.28)
Scain, 2009
-0.40 (-0.92, 0.12)
Schillinger, 2009
0.20 (-0.25, 0.65)
Rosal, 2011
-0.25 (-0.72, 0.22)
Toobert, 2011
0.00 (-0.48, 0.48)
Rygg, 2012
-0.10 (-0.45, 0.25)
Subtotal (I-squared = 37.6%, p = 0.141)
-0.20 (-0.43, 0.02)
Poor
S. A. Brown, 2002
-0.79 (-1.40, -0.18)
A. Philis-Tsimikas, 2011
-0.60 (-1.34, 0.14)
Subtotal (I-squared = 0.0%, p = 0.698)
-0.71 (-1.18, -0.24)
Overall (I-squared = 56.9%, p = 0.013)
-0.23 (-0.44, -0.02)
-2
-1.5
-1
-.5
0
.5
1
← Favors treatment
Favors control →

Return to Contents

Figure 6. Effect of group visits compared to usual care on HbA1C at 7-12 month follow-up, by duration of intervention

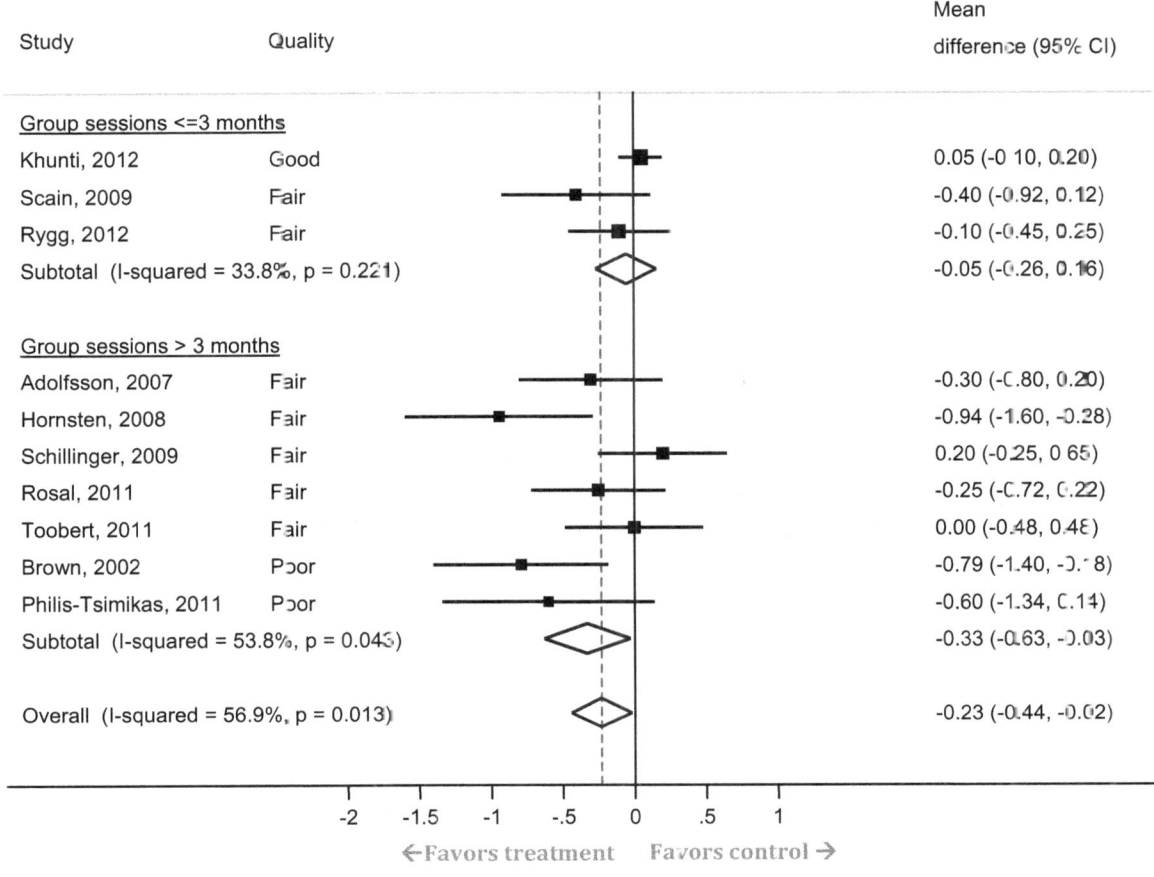

Multiple Chronic Conditions

Four studies evaluated the Chronic Disease Self-Management Program (CDSMP)[61] in populations with various chronic conditions not limited to a particular disease group (Tables 13 and 14).[89-92] The CDSMP was designed as a workshop held in community settings such as senior centers, churches, libraries and hospitals. People with different chronic health problems attend together, meeting 2.5 hours once per week for six to seven weeks. The workshops are facilitated by two trained leaders, one or both of whom are non-health professionals with chronic diseases themselves.

The largest study evaluated the CDSMP in multiple community-based sites in the US and found it was associated with improved health behaviors, including cognitive symptom management, reduced hospital utilization, and improved self-rated health and disability at six months.[92] Of note, the 17 percent of patients who did not complete the study tended to have more illness related disability than those completing the trial, though there was no differential loss to follow-up between the two groups. The authors report that a full intent-to-treat analysis was conducted and that results were similar, but they fully report only the per-protocol analysis. Seventy-two percent of the wait-list control group elected to enroll in the CDSMP after the trial. A pre-post two-year follow-up study of all CDSMP participants found long-term reductions in ER and outpatient visits as well as improved self-efficacy.[93] The authors estimate the cost of the program to be about $70 per participant (in 1999).

A large northern California study of the Spanish-language adaptation of the CDSMP found the intervention improved self-efficacy in the medium- and long-term, as well as decreased ER visits at 4 and 12 months.[91] Another large study in China found medium-term improvements on a cognitive symptom scale, but not in self-efficacy nor on ER visits.[90] Self-efficacy scales also showed mixed findings, with benefits noted in some studies but not in other studies that used the same measures (Table 14). The Dutch study was of poor-quality and found no effect of the intervention on outcomes.[89]

Overall, the peer-led, community-based CDSMP appears to be associated with medium-term improvements in self-efficacy, health status, and health care utilization; and these effects may persist long-term. These findings are based on moderately strong evidence from two large US trials, though findings were not replicated in other countries and the findings likely apply most to patients engaged enough in care to agree to attend a multi-week course.

Return to Contents

Group Visits Focusing on Education for the Management of Chronic Conditions in Adults

Table 13. Characteristics of group visit interventions focusing on education for the management of chronic conditions in populations with multiple disease groups

Study	Sample size Setting *Program name, if applicable*	Demographics: Mean age % male % minority Mean disease duration	GV structure: # Visits, frequency Duration Group size	GV content: SME (self-mgmt) DE (didactic) EE (experiential)	GV leaders: Number of leaders Profession type	Comparator
Lorig, 1999[92]	N=952* US *CDSMP*	Mean age 65 35% male 9.7% non-white Duration NR (heart disease, lung disease, arthritis, and stroke)	7 weekly sessions 7 weeks total 10-15 patients	SME	2 trained peer leaders	Usual care
Lorig, 2003[91]	N=551 US *CDSMP (Spanish)*	Mean age 57 21% male Race NR Duration NR	6 weekly sessions 6 weeks total 10-15 patients	SME	2 trained peer leaders	Usual care
Fu, 2003[90]	N=954 China *CDSMP*	Mean age 64 29% male Race NR Duration NR	7 weekly sessions 7 weeks total Group size NR	SME	2 trained peer volunteer leaders	Usual care
Elzen, 2007[89]	N=136 Netherlands *CDSMP*	Mean age 68 37% male Race NR Duration NR	6 weekly sessions 6 weeks 10-13 patients	SME	2 psychologists or 1 psychologist plus peer leader	Usual care

*N=1,128 in the intent-to-treat analysis. Results are reported as being similar in ITT and per-protocol analysis, but full results reporting only available for the group completing the study.

Group Visits Focusing on Education for the Management of Chronic Conditions in Adults

Table 14. Findings from interventions comparing group visits to usual care control for the management of chronic conditions in studies of populations with multiple disease groups

Study	Outcome measure	Findings by time period*				GV intervention duration	#visits	% Participation† / % Loss Follow-up‡	Study quality
		0-3 mo	4-6 mo	7-12 mo	13+ mo				
Self-efficacy									
Lorig 1999[92]	Cognitive symptom management	NR	+	NR	NR	7 weeks	7	NR / 17	Fair
Lorig, 2003[91]	4-item self-efficacy scale	NR	+	+	NR	6 weeks	6	NR / 51	Fair
Fu, 2003[90]	4-item self-efficacy scale	NR	≈	NR	NR	7 weeks	7	NA / 13	Fair
	Cognitive symptom scale	NR	+	NR	NR				
Elzen, 2007[89]	GSES-16 (Dutch)	≈	≈	NR	NR	6 weeks	6	26 / 10	Poor
	Cognitive symptom scale	≈	≈	NR	NR				
Quality of life									
Lorig, 1999[92]	Self-rated health§	NR	+	NR	NR	7 weeks	7	NR / 17	Fair
	Disability (HAQ)	NR	+	NR	NR				
Elzen, 2007[89]	RAND-36 physical and mental components	≈	≈	NR	NR	6 weeks	6	26 / 10	Poor
Utilization									
Lorig, 1999[92]	Physician visits	NR	≈	NR	NR	7 weeks	7	NR / 17	Fair
	Hospital stays	NR	+	NR	NR				
Lorig, 2003[91]	Physician visits	NR	≈	≈	NR	6 weeks	6	NR / 51	Fair
	ER visits	NR	+	+	NR				
	Hospital days	NR	≈	≈	NR				
Fu, 2003[90]	Physician visits	NR	≈	NR	NR	7 weeks	7	NA / 13	Fair
	ER visits	NR	≈	NR	NR				
	Hospital days	NR	≈	NR	NR				

*Symbols pertain to statistical significance $p<0.05$: ≈ indicates no difference between arms; + indicates in favor of the GV arm; - indicates in favor of the C arm; NR = not reported.
†Defined as percent eligible for enrollment among those invited to participate.
‡Defined as percent lost to follow-up among those randomized.
§National Health Interview Survey measure[94]

Chronic Pain

Four studies evaluated the effects of group-based interventions compared to usual care,[95,96] educational reading materials,[97] or individual treatment[98] in patients with chronic pain (Tables 15-17). Providers for the group-based interventions varied, and included psychologists, physicians, rehabilitation specialists, nurses, physiotherapists, and physical therapists. All of the studies examined group interventions with self-management skills education components. The group-based interventions ranged from 7 to 12 sessions conducted weekly or every-other-week, and most included approximately six patients per group. Length of follow-up for the studies was generally short, approximately 0 to 3 months following completion of the group, however, two studies evaluated some outcomes up to a year following intervention completion. Though many findings from the studies were not statistically significant and did not differ from the comparison, some results favored the group-based interventions. The studies all reported results from multiple outcome measures.

Ersek and colleagues reported similar effects of a group-based intervention and educational reading materials on functional status and self-efficacy measures at three months.[97] Gustavsson and colleagues (2010) reported that compared to usual individual physical therapy care, a group-based intervention had largely similar effects on multiple measures of pain control and self-efficacy, but was associated with more improvement on the Neck Disability Index and the Coping Strategies Questionnaire at 20 weeks of follow-up.[98] The group visits intervention group also reported using less medication for pain at 20 weeks. One poor-quality study found group self-management education was associated with improved pain scores, reduction in psychological distress, and decreased self-reported physician visits compared to a usual care control group over 12 months. However, numerous methodological flaws including marked differences in follow-up rates between groups limit confidence in these results.[28,95] Finally, a paper by Vlaeyen and colleagues (1996) describes two group-based interventions (only one including an SME component) compared to each other and to a waitlist control group.[96] They report no significant differences between the group-based interventions at 6 and 12 month follow-up on almost all of the 12 outcome variables included, but report that both group-based conditions showed a benefit over waitlist control on about half of the outcomes (knowledge, pain coping, pain control, relaxation, pain behavior, and fear).

Overall, a very small body of literature suggests group-based self-management education interventions may improve pain coping skills at least over the short-term, though the strength of this evidence is low because there were few studies and the methodological quality of one of the studies finding benefit was poor.

Return to Contents

Group Visits Focusing on Education for the Management of Chronic Conditions in Adults

Table 15. Characteristics of group visit interventions focusing on education for the management of chronic pain

Study	Sample size Setting *Program name, if applicable*	Demographics: Mean age % male % minority Mean disease duration	GV structure: # Visits, frequency Duration Group size	GV content: SME (self-mgmt) DE (didactic) EE (experiential)	GV leaders: Number of leaders Profession type	Comparator
Chronic Pain						
Ersek, 2003[97]	N=45 US	Age 81.9 Gender 13% Race 84.71% Caucasian Duration NR	7 weekly sessions 8 weeks 3-8 patients	SME	2 leaders Doctoral-level health providers	Receipt of an educational booklet on pain
Gustavsson, 2010[98]	N=156 Sweden *PASS*	Age 45.7 Gender 11% Race NR Duration NR	7 weekly sessions 7 weeks + 1 booster at week 20 Group size NR	SME, EE	1 leader Physical therapists	Individual physical therapy sessions
Haugli, 2000 & Haugli, 2003[28,95]	N=174 Norway	Age 43.08 Gender 2.27% Race NR Duration 9.89 years	12 every-other-week sessions 9 months (including a summer break) 6-10 patients	SME	2 leaders Nurses, physicians physiotherapists	Usual care
Vlaeyen, 1996[96]	N=131 Netherlands	Age 44 Gender 12% Race NR Duration 10.2 years	12 sessions 6 weeks Maximum of 6 patients	GV1: SME, EE GV2: DE, EE	Rehabilitation staff, psychologist	Usual care

Group Visits Focusing on Education for the Management of Chronic Conditions in Adults

Table 16. Findings from interventions comparing group visits to control for the management of chronic pain

Study	Outcome	Findings by time period*				GV duration	#visits	% Participation†/ % Loss Follow-up‡	Study quality
		0-3 mo	4-6 mo	7-12 mo	13+ mo				
Self-efficacy									
Ersek, 2003[97]	Survey of Pain Attitudes	≈	NR	NR	NR	8 weeks	7	NA / 13	Fair
Gustavsson, 2010[98]	CSQ (pain control)	+	NR	NR	NR	20 weeks	8	84 / 20	Good
	Self Efficacy Scale	≈	NR	NR	NR	20 weeks			
Vlaeyen, 1996[96] GV1 vs. UC	Pain coping construct	+	NR	NR	NR	6 weeks	12	NR / 20	Fair
Vlaeyen, 1996[96] GV2 vs. UC	Pain coping construct	+	NR	NR	NR				
Quality of life									
Ersek, 2003[97]	SF-36 (physical and physical functioning)	≈	NR	NR	NR	8 weeks	7	NA / 13	Fair
	Graded chronic pain scale – activity interference	≈							
Haugli, 2000 & Haugli, 2003[28,95]	VAS (pain)	≈	NR	+§	NR	9 months	12	NA / 33	Poor
Gustavsson, 2010[98]	Neck Disability Index	+	NR	NR	NR	20 weeks	8	84 / 20	Good
Utilization/Costs									
Haugli, 2000 & Haugli, 2003[28,95]	Self-reported MD visits	+	NR	+§	NR	9 months	12	NA / 33	Poor

*Symbols pertain to statistical significance p<0.05; ≈ indicates no difference between arms, + indicates in favor of the GV arm; - indicates in favor of the C arm; NR = not reported.
†Defined as percent eligible for enrollment among those invited to participate.
‡Defined as percent lost to follow-up among those randomized.
§P-value not reported.

Table 17. Summary of findings from head-to-head group visit interventions and group vs. individual visit interventions for the management of chronic pain

Study	Arm 1	Arm 2	Key findings
Chronic Pain			
Ersek, 2003[97]	GV (7 SME sessions)	Educational booklet on pain	There was a significant improvement in physical role functioning and in pain intensity directly following treatment, but not 3 months after treatment, though no significant effect was noted for other primary outcome variables including physical functioning, activity interference, and depression.
Vlaeyen, 1996[96]	GV (12 SME, EE, DE sessions)	GV (12 DE, EE sessions)	Significant improvement of knowledge, pain coping, pain control, and relaxation for both GV groups compared to control at immediate follow-up; non-significant differences between GV groups at 6 and 12-month follow-up on all primary outcomes.
Gustavsson, 2010[98]	GV (8 session, SME, EE)	Individual physical therapy	GV was positively associated with most assessed outcomes including pain coping, pain control, catastrophizing, pain scores, and anxiety, though effects on depression were non-significant.

DISCUSSION

We found 79 trials examining the effects of group visit interventions across a variety of chronic illnesses. Despite the large evidence base, it is difficult to draw overall conclusions about the effectiveness of group visit interventions in patients with chronic illness in part because of the diversity of patient populations studied, interventions tested and outcomes reported. Nevertheless, in general, many group visit interventions appear to be able to improve short- and medium-term patient self-efficacy, but there was little consistent, fair-to-good quality evidence that they improved quality of life, health outcomes, or health care utilization. We found that diabetes group visit interventions were likely associated with small short-term improvements in glycemic control. The longer-term effects of group visit interventions are largely unknown since the vast majority of studies focused on short-term effects.

As the description of studies in our review suggests, educating patients with chronic illness is a highly complex endeavor with interventions varying in their intended purpose, content delivered, leadership, intensity, format and more. Studies comparing two or more active interventions can begin to help elucidate whether or not there are certain intervention factors associated with better outcomes. There were few studies directly comparing a purely didactic, informational education approach to one focused on core self-management skills, though, not surprisingly, most studies finding improvements in self-efficacy focused on the latter. Group and individual approaches to education appear to have similar effects. Other comparisons are summarized in the tables above, but there were not enough studies to draw conclusions about the effects of other intervention elements.

Learning and mastering chronic illness self-management is a time-consuming process. Theoretically, one might reasonably expect the duration of an intervention to be associated with its effectiveness, but we found it difficult to confirm this hypothesis. For example, we did find greater improvement in glycemic control among those interventions lasting longer than 3 months compared to interventions of shorter duration. However, the interventions of longer duration were also of lower methodological quality. Unfortunately, we found few studies examining the effects of a "booster" session (i.e., a refresher session conducted some time after the initial intervention ended).

It is unclear why the group visit interventions literature has not found a consistent impact on health, utilization, or quality of life outcomes despite the logical inference that improved self-efficacy and self-management skills should lead to improved self-management, improved disease control and coping, and resultant improved outcomes. It is possible that intervention or follow-up duration has been inadequate as discussed above. It is also possible that - in an era promoting guideline dissemination, electronic health records, and quality improvement - it is becoming increasingly difficult to demonstrate incremental benefits of an educational intervention because usual care has improved over time. Indeed, a recent trial of intensive diabetes treatment found few health outcome effects in part, as the authors speculate, because treatment in the usual care group was quite good.[99]

We found no formal cost-effectiveness data to guide decision-making about the wisdom of widespread investment in group visit education modalities. However, one can easily infer that there is likely to be great variation in costs of different interventions depending on the personnel leading the visits, the duration of the intervention, and the number of visits. For example, some interventions – such as cognitive behavioral therapy – are fairly intensive and would involve allocating a professional's time. Many of the self-management skills training interventions improved self-efficacy but not health outcomes. Whether group visit expenditures are warranted may depend on how highly more proximate outcome measures like self-efficacy are valued by patients and the health system.

On the other hand, peer-led, community-based self-management programs – such as the CDSMP – may represent a low-cost way of improving self-efficacy and perhaps improving other outcomes. However, such programs do not provide some of the core skills and information patients with a given chronic illness might need to help self-manage their illness (e.g., glucose self-monitoring, dietary plans, CHF management plans). It is not clear from most studies how this core information was provided. If VA were to implement such peer-led self-management programs, it would likely still need a structure for providing basic disease-specific informational needs, though this could be accomplished in different ways including single group visit, educational pamphlets, etc. It is also not clear how much the community-based nature of the intervention matters. Offering the programs in local churches, and community centers may make it easier for patients to participate on an ongoing basis and perhaps may provide a less threatening environment. It would be useful to use qualitative and formative evaluation methods if implementation of such programs were considered, in order to shed more light on such issues.

Although we did not find direct harms associated with group visits, the lack of robust findings that group visits improve long-term health outcomes invites caution around blanket recommendations for widespread and rapid group visit implementation. This is especially true for patient populations with specific health needs. For instance, travel and participation time involved in getting to and participating in group visits may preclude participation for patients with limited work schedule flexibility, and may be prohibitive for frail, older participants.

Of note, we excluded studies focused on experiential exercise (i.e., group exercise classes) without a distinct educational component, so we cannot comment on their effectiveness. Other reviews may provide more information on the utility of experiential exercise sessions [2,3] We found few studies examining the incremental benefits of experiential exercise added to group education, so were unable to draw conclusions about the utility of such interventions.

GENERALIZABILITY

Participation rates, when reported, ranged from 13 to 100 percent though many studies provided little information about the recruitment process. The broad range of participation, in part, reflects the many levels of potential eligibility, and the higher rates may be misleading. For instance, in one study, over 21,000 patients were identified in an administrative database.[57] Only one-third of these patients were successfully contacted by letter, only one-quarter of who were screened by phone, and then only a small portion of these patients attended in-person screening. Though 91 percent of those eligible at this stage were randomized, only one percent of patients identified through the administrative database actually enrolled in the study. In practical terms, these studies generally represent a small fraction of the total number of patients with chronic illness and, therefore, will apply to relatively few people identified through patient registries Findings from the studies included in this review are likely to be most applicable to those patients who are easy to contact, have time to participate in an intervention, and who have enough motivation to enter into a study in the first place.

We identified four studies that examined group visit interventions in Veteran populations, one each in hypertensive,[62] congestive heart failure,[59] chronic obstructive pulmonary disease,[57] and diabetes populations.[80] These studies investigated interventions that were similar to other interventions tested in non-Veteran populations. We found no studies evaluating interventions that were specific to a given setting (e.g., tied to a specific technology unavailable in VA) or that would not be potentially feasible in a VA setting.

LIMITATIONS

In setting out to perform this systematic review of group visit interventions led by non-prescribing facilitators, a chief limitation is comparability of studies given the vast heterogeneity and complexity of intervention content and outcomes examined. Although there have been many published studies testing group visit effectiveness, we found few with similar enough characteristics to be explicitly compared in meta-analyses. The sheer number and variety of outcomes reported across studies precluded reporting of all outcomes. We prespecified those outcomes that were either likely to be commonly reported, represented clinically important outcomes, or measured self-efficacy since this was, in many cases, the intended effect of the intervention. We acknowledge, however, that there may be other important outcomes not captured in this report. Most notably, we did not consider knowledge improvement outcomes. Many studies reported various knowledge outcomes, but few were standardized and they varied so broadly that any comparison across studies would have been impossible. Moreover, one could argue the clinical importance of short-term knowledge gains if they do not translate into gains in self-efficacy, health outcomes, or quality of life. Additionally, we found good quality trials testing the effectiveness of multicomponent interventions that included both, group and individual elements.[100] Unfortunately, these trials were not included in our review because the independent effects of the group visit component could not be evaluated.

Return to Contents

FUTURE RESEARCH

We identify gaps in evidence of the effectiveness of group visit interventions in Table 18.

Table 18. Evidence gaps and future research

Evidence Gap	Recommendations / Types of studies to consider
Patients/Populations	
Low participation of eligible study participants and high attrition of randomized participants. Few good quality studies in patients with asthma, COPD, CHF, chronic pain, and multiple chronic conditions.	Better reporting of recruitment population and improved recruitment and retention practices. More trials in these populations.
Interventions	
Lack of clarity as to which intervention components are important in achieving improvements. Few studies of group interventions using modern technologies such as mobile platforms and video-based interventions.	Head-to-head comparative trials. More trials of interventions using technologies allowing remote participation. Studies assessing whether use of such technologies to deliver interventions improves participation and retention rates.
Comparator	
Relatively few studies with active comparison groups.	Comparative effectiveness trials. For example, studies showing that mailed and phone-based self-management education programs were as effective as in-person group visits are interesting and point to alternative educational forums that may appeal to patients with time or geographic constraints. Also, more studies comparing individual to group-based education could better clarify the relative merits of each approach.
Outcomes	
Studies evaluated dozens of different outcomes, many of which were non-standardized metrics of uncertain validity	Standardized approach to outcome measurement and use of well validated scales.
Timing	
Lack of studies examining long-term outcomes. Few trials assessed the effects of booster sessions.	Trials with longer-term follow-up. Trials evaluating the effects and timing of booster sessions.
Setting	
Few trials in community and rural settings	Test telehealth trials of group visits and trials located in community settings such as churches and community centers.

CONCLUSION

A large number of studies have evaluated group visit interventions in a variety of patient populations. Intervention characteristics and effects differed depending on the chronic illness in which they were studied. Overall, group visits have the potential to improve patient self-efficacy, though there is little consistent data that they improve health, utilization, or quality of life outcomes. Group visits may be as effective as individual education visits and may represent a reasonable alternative for educating patients with chronic illness, though the varied and sometimes low participation and retention rates suggest they should not be the sole alternative.

REFERENCES

1. Edelman D, McDuffie JR, Oddone E, Gierisch JM, Nagi A, Williams JW, Jr. Shared Medical Appointments for Chronic Medical Conditions: A Systematic Review. *VAESP Project #09-010.* 2012.

2. Han A, Judd M, Welch V, Wu T, Tugwell P, Wells GA. Tai chi for treating rheumatoid arthritis. *Cochrane Database of Systematic Reviews.* 2010;7:7.

3. Ashworth NL, Chad KE, Harrison EL, Reeder BA, Marshall SC. Home versus center based physical activity programs in older adults. *Cochrane Database of Systematic Reviews.* 2009;1:1.

4. Anonymous. Effect of intensive blood-glucose control with metformin on complications in overweight patients with type 2 diabetes (UKPDS 34). UK Prospective Diabetes Study (UKPDS) Group. *Lancet.* 1998;352(9131):854-865.

5. Harris RP, Helfand M, Woolf SH, et al. Current methods of the US Preventive Services Task Force. A review of the process. *Am. J. Prev. Med.* 2001;30(3S):21-35.

6. Guyatt G, Oxman AD, Akl EA, et al. GRADE guidelines: 1. Introduction-GRADE evidence profiles and summary of findings tables. *J. Clin. Epidemiol.* 2011;64(4):383-394.

7. Lorig K, Stewart A, Ritter P, González V, Laurent D, Lynch J. Outcome Measures for Health Education and other Health Care Interventions. Thousand Oaks CA: Sage Publications. 1996. pp 24-25, 41-45.

8. Hibbard JH, Stockard J, Mahoney ER, Tusler M. Development of the Patient Activation Measure (PAM): Conceptualizing and Measuring Activation in Patients and Consumers. *Health Services Research August.* 2004;39(4, Part I):1005-1026.

9. Greene J, Hibbard JH. Why Does Patient Activation Matter? An Examination of the Relationships Between Patient Activation and Health-Related Outcomes. *J. Gen. Intern. Med.* 2012;27(5):520-526.

10. DerSimonian R, Laird N. Meta-analysis in clinical trials. *Control. Clin. Trials.* Sep 1986;7(3):177-188.

11. Higgins JPT, Altman DG, editors. Chapter 8: Assessing risk of bias in included studies. In: Higgins JPT, Green S (editors). *Cochrane Handbook for Systematic Reviews of Interventions.* 2008;Version 5.0.1. The Cochrane Collaboration, 2008. Availablefrom www.cochrane-handbook.org.

12. Egger M, Davey Smith G, Schneider M, Minder C. Bias in meta-analysis detected by a simple, graphical test. *BMJ.* Sep 13 1997;315(7109):629-634.

13. D'Eramo Melkus G, Chyun D, Vorderstrasse A, Newlin K, Jefferson V, Langerman S. The effect of a diabetes education, coping skills training, and care intervention on physiological and psychosocial outcomes in black women with type 2 diabetes. *Biol Res Nurs.* Jul 2010;12(1):7-19.

14. Weinger K, Beverly EA, Lee Y, Sitnokov L, Ganda OP, Caballero AE. The effect of a structured behavioral intervention on poorly controlled diabetes: a randomized controlled trial. *Arch. Intern. Med.* Dec 12 2011;171(22):1990-1999.

15. Brown SA, Garcia AA, Kouzekanani K, Hanis CL. Culturally competent diabetes self-management education for Mexican Americans: the Starr County border health initiative. *Diabetes Care.* Feb 2002;25(2):259-268.

16. Brown SA, Blozis SA, Kouzekanani K, Garcia AA, Winchell M, Hanis CL. Dosage effects of diabetes self-management education for Mexican Americans: the Starr County Border Health Initiative. *Diabetes Care.* Mar 2005;28(3):527-532.

17. Hornsten A, Stenlund H, Lundman B, Sandstrom H. Improvements in HbA1c remain after 5 years--a follow up of an educational intervention focusing on patients' personal understandings of type 2 diabetes. *Diabetes Res. Clin. Pract.* Jul 2008;81(1):50-55.

18. Philis-Tsimikas A, Fortmann A, Lleva-Ocana L, Walker C, Gallo LC. Peer-led diabetes education programs in high-risk Mexican Americans improve glycemic control compared with standard approaches: a Project Dulce promotora randomized trial. *Diabetes Care.* Sep 2011;34(9):1926-1931.

19. Rosal MC, Ockene IS, Restrepo A, et al. Randomized trial of a literacy-sensitive, culturally tailored diabetes self-management intervention for low-income latinos: latinos en control. *Diabetes Care.* Apr 2011;34(4):838-844.

20. Surwit RS, van Tilburg MA, Zucker N, et al. Stress management improves long-term glycemic control in type 2 diabetes. *Diabetes Care.* Vol 252002:30-34.

21. Rygg LO, Rise MB, Gronning K, Steinsbekk A. Efficacy of ongoing group based diabetes self-management education for patients with type 2 diabetes mellitus. A randomised controlled trial. *Patient Educ. Couns.* Jan 2012;86(1):98-105.

22. Ettinger WH, Jr., Burns R, Messier SP, et al. A randomized trial comparing aerobic exercise and resistance exercise with a health education program in older adults with knee osteoarthritis. The Fitness Arthritis and Seniors Trial (FAST). *JAMA.* Jan 1 1997;277(1):25-31.

23. Hammond A, Lincoln N, Sutcliffe L. A crossover trial evaluating an educational-behavioural joint protection programme for people with rheumatoid arthritis. *Patient Educ. Couns.* May 1999;37(1):19-32.

24. Clemson L, Cumming RG, Kendig H, Swann M, Heard R, Taylor K. The effectiveness of a community-based program for reducing the incidence of falls in the elderly: a randomized trial. *J. Am. Geriatr. Soc.* Sep 2004;52(9):1487-1494.

25. Shumway-Cook A, Silver HF, LeMier M, York S, Cummings P, Koepsell TD. Effectiveness of a community-based multifactorial intervention on falls and fall risk factors in community-living older adults: a randomized, controlled trial. *Journals of Gerontology Series A: Biological Sciences & Medical Sciences.* 2007;62A(12):1420-1427.

26. Svetkey LP, Pollak KI, Yancy WS, Jr., et al. Hypertension improvement project: randomized trial of quality improvement for physicians and lifestyle modification for patients. *Hypertension.* Dec 2009;54(6):1226-1233.

27. Smeulders ES, van Haastregt JC, Ambergen T, et al. Heart failure patients with a lower educational level and better cognitive status benefit most from a self-management group programme. *Patient Educ. Couns.* Nov 2010;81(2):214-221.

28. Haugli L, Steen E, Laerum E, Finset A, Nygaard R. Agency orientation and chronic musculoskeletal pain: effects of a group learning program based on the personal construct theory. *Clin. J. Pain.* Dec 2000;16(4):281-289.

29. Lorig KR, Ritter PL, Laurent DD, Fries JF. Long-term randomized controlled trials of tailored-print and small-group arthritis self-management interventions. *Med. Care.* Apr 2004;42(4):346-354.

30. Schillinger D, Handley M, Wang F, Hammer H. Effects of self-management support on structure, process, and outcomes among vulnerable patients with diabetes: a three-arm practical clinical trial. *Diabetes Care.* Apr 2009;32(4):559-566.

31. Ackerman IN, Buchbinder R, Osborne RH. Challenges in Evaluating an Arthritis Self-management Program for People with Hip and Knee Osteoarthritis in Real-world Clinical Settings. *The Journal of Rheumatology.* 2012;39(5):1-9.

32. Barlow JH, Turner AP, Wright CC. A randomized controlled study of the Arthritis Self-Management Programme in the UK. *Health Educ. Res.* Dec 2000;15(6):665-680.

33. Breedland I, van Scheppingen C, Leijsma M, Verheij-Jansen NP, van Weert E. Effects of a group-based exercise and educational program on physical performance and disease self-management in rheumatoid arthritis: a randomized controlled study. *Phys. Ther.* Jun 2011;91(6):879-893.

34. Buszewicz M, Rait G, Griffin M, et al. Self management of arthritis in primary care: randomised controlled trial. *BMJ (Clinical research ed.).* Oct 2006;333(7574):879.

35. Patel A, Buszewicz M, Beecham J, et al. Economic evaluation of arthritis self management in primary care. *BMJ.* 2009;339:b3532.

36. Freeman K, Hammond A, Lincoln NB. Use of cognitive-behavioural arthritis education programmes in newly diagnosed rheumatoid arthritis. *Clin. Rehabil.* Dec 2002;16(8):828-836.

37. Giraudet-Le Quintrec J, Mayoux-Benhamou A, Ravaud P, et al. Effect of a collective educational program for patients with rheumatoid arthritis: a prospective 12-month randomized controlled trial. *J. Rheumatol.* 2007;34(8):1684-1691.

38. Hewlett S, Ambler N, Almeida C, et al. Self-management of fatigue in rheumatoid arthritis: a randomised controlled trial of group cognitive-behavioural therapy. *Ann. Rheum. Dis.* Jun 2011;70(6):1060-1067.

39. Kaplan S, Kozin F. A controlled study of group counseling in rheumatoid arthritis. *J. Rheumatol.* Jan-Feb 1981;8(1):91-99.

40. Lorig K, Lubeck D, Kraines RG, Seleznick M, Holman HR. Outcomes of self-help education for patients with arthritis. *Arthritis Rheum.* Jun 1985;28(6):680-685.

41. Lorig K, Gonzalez VM, Ritter P. Community-based Spanish language arthritis education program: a randomized trial. *Med. Care.* Sep 1999;37(9):957-963.

42. Riemsma RP, Taal E, Rasker JJ. Group education for patients with rheumatoid arthritis and their partners. *Arthritis Rheum.* Aug 15 2003;49(4):556-566.

43. Sevick MA, Miller GD, Loeser RF, Williamson JD, Messier SP. Cost-effectiveness of exercise and diet in overweight and obese adults with knee osteoarthritis. *Med. Sci. Sports Exerc.* 2009;41(6):1167-1174.

44. Taal E, Riemsma RP, Brus HL, Seydel ER, Rasker JJ, Wiegman O. Group education for patients with rheumatoid arthritis. *Patient Educ. Couns.* May 1993;20(2-3):177-187.

45. Arnold CM, Faulkner RA. The effect of aquatic exercise and education on lowering fall risk in older adults with hip osteoarthritis. *J Aging Phys Act.* Jul 2010;18(3):245-260.

46. Ryan JW, Spellbring AM. Implementing strategies to decrease risk of falls in older women. *J. Gerontol. Nurs.* Dec 1996;22(12):25-31.

47. Hammond A, Bryan J, Hardy A. Effects of a modular behavioural arthritis education programme: a pragmatic parallel-group randomized controlled trial. *Rheumatology (Oxford).* Nov 2008;47(11):1712-1718.

48. Wilson SR, Scamagas P, German DF, et al. A controlled trial of two forms of self-management education for adults with asthma. *The American journal of medicine.* Jun 1993;94(6):564-576.

49. Abdulwadud O, Abramson M, Forbes A, James A, Walters EH. Evaluation of a randomised controlled trial of adult asthma education in a hospital setting. *Thorax.* Jun 1999;54(6):493-500.

50. Allen RM, Jones MP, Oldenburg B. Randomised trial of an asthma self-management programme for adults. *Thorax.* Jul 1995;50(7):731-738.

51. Bolton MB, Tilley BC, Kuder J, Reeves T, Schultz LR. The cost and effectiveness of an education program for adults who have asthma. *J. Gen. Intern. Med.* Sep-Oct 1991;6(5):401-407.

52. Snyder SE, Winder JA, Creer TJ. Development and evaluation of an adult asthma self-management program: Wheezers Anonymous. *J. Asthma.* 1987;24(3):153-158.

53. Wilson JS, Fitzsimons D, Bradbury I, Stuart Elborn J. Does additional support by nurses enhance the effect of a brief smoking cessation intervention in people with moderate to severe chronic obstructive pulmonary disease? A randomised controlled trial. *Int. J. Nurs. Stud.* Apr 2008;45(4):508-517.

54. Bestall JC, Paul EA, Garrod R, Garnham R, Jones RW, Wedzicha AJ. Longitudinal trends in exercise capacity and health status after pulmonary rehabilitation in patients with COPD. *Respir. Med.* Feb 2003;97(2):173-180.

55. Effing T, Zielhuis G, Kerstjens H, van der Valk P, van der Palen J. Community based physiotherapeutic exercise in COPD self-management: a randomised controlled trial. *Respir. Med.* Mar 2011;105(3):418-426.

56. Ninot G, Moullec G, Picot MC, et al. Cost-saving effect of supervised exercise associated to COPD self-management education program. *Respir. Med.* Mar 2011;105(3):377-385.

57. Kunik ME, Veazey C, Cully JA, et al. COPD education and cognitive behavioral therapy group treatment for clinically significant symptoms of depression and anxiety in COPD patients: a randomized controlled trial. *Psychol. Med.* Mar 2008;38(3):385-396.

58. Moore SM, Charvat JM, Gordon NH, et al. Effects of a CHANGE intervention to increase exercise maintenance following cardiac events. *nn. Behav. Med.* 2006;31(1):53-62.

59. Chang BH, Hendricks A, Zhao Y, Rothendler JA, LoCastro JS, Slawsky MT. A relaxation response randomized trial on patients with chronic heart failure. *J Cardiopulm Rehabil.* May-Jun 2005;25(3):149-157.

60. Smeulders ES, van Haastregt JC, Ambergen T, et al. Nurse-led self-management group programme for patients with congestive heart failure: randomized controlled trial. *J. Adv. Nurs.* Jul 2010;66(7):1487-1499.

61. Stanford School of Medicine. Chronic Disease Self-Management Program. http://patienteducation.stanford.edu/programs/cdsmp.html. Accessed on Sept. 20, 2012.

62. Nessman DG, Carnahan JE, Nugent CA. Increasing compliance. Patient-operated hypertension groups. *Arch. Intern. Med.* Nov 1980;140(11):1427-1430.

63. Rujiwatthanakorn D, Panpakdee O, Malathum P, Tanomsup S. Effectiveness of a self-management program for Thais with essential hypertension. *Pacific Rim International Journal of Nursing Research.* 2011;15(2):97-109.

64. Balcazar HG, Byrd TL, Ortiz M, Tondapu SR, Chavez M. A randomized community intervention to improve hypertension control among Mexican Americans: using the promotoras de salud community outreach model. *J. Health Care Poor Underserved.* Nov 2009;20(4):1079-1094.

65. Figar S, Galarza C, Petrlik E, et al. Effect of education on blood pressure control in elderly persons: a randomized controlled trial. *Am. J. Hypertens.* Jul 2006;19(7):737-743.

66. Scala D, D'Avino M, Cozzolino S, et al. Promotion of behavioural change in people with hypertension: an intervention study. *Pharm. World Sci.* Dec 2008;30(6):834-839.

67. Baghianimoghadam MH, Rahaee Z, Morowatisharifabad MA, Sharifirad G, Andishmand A, Azadbakht L. Effects of education on self-monitoring of blood pressure based on BASNEF model in hypertensive patients. *JRMS.* 2010;15(2):70-77.

68. Khunti K, Gray LJ, Skinner T, et al. Effectiveness of a diabetes education and self management programme (DESMOND) for people with newly diagnosed type 2 diabetes mellitus: three year follow-up of a cluster randomised controlled trial in primary care. *BMJ.* 2012;344(e2333).

69. Lorig K, Ritter PL, Villa FJ, Armas J. Community-based peer-led diabetes self-management: a randomized trial. *Diabetes Educ.* Jul-Aug 2009;35(4):641-651.

70. Davies MJ, Heller S, Skinner TC, et al. Effectiveness of the diabetes education and self management for ongoing and newly diagnosed (DESMOND) programme for people with newly diagnosed type 2 diabetes: cluster randomised controlled trial. *BMJ* Mar 1 2008;336(7642):491-495.

71. Deakin TA, Cade JE, Williams R, Greenwood DC. Structured patient education: the diabetes X-PERT Programme makes a difference. *Diabet Med.* Vol 23. 2006/08/23 ed2006:944-954

72. Kulzer B, Hermanns N, Reinecker H, Haak T. Effects of self-management training in Type 2 diabetes: a randomized, prospective trial. *Diabet. Med.* Apr 2007;24(4):415-423.

73. De Greef K, Deforche B, Tudor-Locke C, De Bourdeaudhuij I. Increasing physical activity in Belgian type 2 diabetes patients: a three-arm randomized controlled trial. *Int J Behav Med.* Vol 18. 2010/11/06 ed2011:188-198.

74. Rickheim PL, Weaver TW, Flader JL, Kendall DM. Assessment of group versus individual diabetes education: a randomized study. *Diabetes Care.* Vol 25. 2002/01/30 ed2002:269-274.

75. Adolfsson ET, Walker-Engstrom ML, Smide B, Wikblad K. Patient education in type 2 diabetes: a randomized controlled 1-year follow-up study. *Diabetes Res. Clin. Pract.* Jun 2007;76(3):341-350.

76. Anderson RM, Funnell MM, Nwankwo R, Gillard ML, Oh M, Fitzgerald JT. Evaluating a problem-based empowerment program for African Americans with diabetes: results of a randomized controlled trial. *Ethn. Dis.* Autumn 2005;15(4):671-678.

77. Dejesus RS, Chaudhry R, Leutink DJ, Hinton MA, Cha SS, Stroebel RJ. Effects of efforts to intensify management on blood pressure control among patients with type 2 diabetes mellitus and hypertension: a pilot study. *Vasc Health Risk Manag.* 2009;5:705-711.

78. Lujan J, Ostwald SK, Ortiz M. Promotora diabetes intervention for Mexican Americans. *Diabetes Educ.* Jul-Aug 2007;33(4):660-670.

79. Miller CK, Edwards L, Kissling G, Sanville L. Nutrition education improves metabolic outcomes among older adults with diabetes mellitus: results from a randomized controlled trial. *Preventive Medicine.* Vol 342002:252-259.

80. Raji A, Gomes H, Beard JO, MacDonald P, Conlin PR. A randomized trial comparing intensive and passive education in patients with diabetes mellitus. *Arch. Intern. Med.* Jun 10 2002;162(11):1301-1304.

81. Sarkadi A, Rosenqvist U. Experience-based group education in Type 2 diabetes: a randomised controlled trial. *Patient Educ. Couns.* Jun 2004;53(3):291-298.

82. Scain SF, Friedman R, Gross JL. A structured educational program improves metabolic control in patients with type 2 diabetes: a randomized controlled trial. *Diabetes Educ.* Jul-Aug 2009;35(4):603-611.

83. Sharifirad G, Najimi A, Hassanzadeh A, Azadbakht L. Does nutrition education improve the risk factors of cardiovascular diseases among elderly with type 2 diabetes? A randomized controlled trial based on an educational model. *J Diabetes.* Apr 28 2012.

84. Sperl-Hillen J, Beaton S, Fernandes O, et al. Comparative effectiveness of patient education methods for type 2 diabetes: a randomized controlled trial. *Arch. Intern. Med.* Dec 12 2011;171(22):2001-2010.

85. Steed L, Lankester J, Barnard M, Earle K, Hurel S, Newman S. Evaluation of the UCL diabetes self-management programme (UCL-DSMP): a randomized controlled trial. *J Health Psychol.* Mar 2005;10(2):261-276.

86. Toobert DJ, Strycker LA, Barrera M, Jr., Osuna D, King DK, Glasgow RE. Outcomes from a multiple risk factor diabetes self-management trial for Latinas: inverted exclamation markViva Bien! *nn. Behav. Med.* Jun 2011;41(3):310-323.

87. Toobert DJ, Strycker LA, King DK, Barrera M, Jr., Osuna D, Glasgow RE. Long-term outcomes from a multiple-risk-factor diabetes trial for Latinas: inverted exclamation markViva Bien! *Transl Behav Med.* Sep 2011;1(3):416-426.

88. Zapotoczky H, Semlitsch B, Herzog G, et al. A controlled study of weight reduction in type 2 diabetics treated by two reinforcers. *International Journal of Behavioral Medicine.* 2001;8(1):42-49.

89. Elzen H, Slaets JP, Snijders TA, Steverink N. Evaluation of the chronic disease self-management program (CDSMP) among chronically ill older people in the Netherlands. *Soc. Sci. Med.* May 2007;64(9):1832-1841.

90. Fu D, Fu H, McGowan P, et al. Implementation and quantitative evaluation of chronic disease self-management programme in Shanghai, China: randomized controlled trial. *Bull. World Health Organ.* 2003;81(3):174-182.

91. Lorig KR, Ritter PL, Gonzalez VM. Hispanic Chronic Disease Self-Management: A Randomized Community-Based Outcome Trial. *Nurs. Res.* Nov-Dec 2003;52(6):361-369.

92. Lorig KR, Sobel DS, Stewart AL, et al. Evidence Suggesting That a Chronic Disease Self-Management Program Can Improve Health Status While Reducing Hospitalization: A Randomized Trial. *Medical Care January.* 1999;37(1):5-14.

93. Lorig KR, Ritter PP, Stewart AL, et al. Chronic Disease Self-Management Program: 2-Year Health Status and Health Care Utilization Outcomes. *Medical Care November.* 2001;39(11):1217-1223.

94. US Department of Commerce. National Health Interview Survey. Bureau of the Census. 1985.

95. Haugli L, Steen E, Laerum E, Nygard R, Finset A. Psychological distress and employment status. Effects of a group learning programme for patients with chronic musculoskeletal pain. *Psychology, Health & Medicine.* May 2003;8(2):135-148.

96. Vlaeyen JW, Teeken-Gruben NJ, Goossens ME, et al. Cognitive-educational treatment of fibromyalgia: a randomized clinical trial. I. Clinical effects. *J. Rheumatol.* Jul 1996;23(7):1237-1245.

97. Ersek M, Turner JA, McCurry SM, Gibbons L, Kraybill BM. Efficacy of a self-management group intervention for elderly persons with chronic pain. *Clin. J. Pain.* May-Jun 2003;19(3):156-167.

98. Gustavsson C, Denison E, von Koch L. Self-management of persistent neck pain: A randomized controlled trial of a multi-component group intervention in primary health care. *European Journal of Pain.* Jul 2010;14(6):e1-e11.

99. Griffin SJ, Borch-Johnsen K, Davies MJ, et al. Effect of early intensive multifactorial therapy on 5-year cardiovascular outcomes in individuals with type 2 diabetes detected by screening (ADDITION-Europe): a cluster-randomised trial. *Lancet.* 9786;378(9786):156-167.

100. Appel LJ, Champagne CM, Harsha DW, et al. Effects of comprehensive lifestyle modification on blood pressure control: main results of the PREMIER clinical trial. *JAMA.* Apr 23-30 2003;289(16):2083-2093.

101. Kritikos V, Armour CL, Bosnic-Anticevich SZ. Interactive small-group asthma education in the community pharmacy setting: a pilot study. *J. Asthma.* Jan-Feb 2007;44(1):57-64.

102. Donesky-Cuenco D, Nguyen HQ, Paul S, Carrieri-Kohlman V. Yoga therapy decreases dyspnea-related distress and improves functional performance in people with chronic obstructive pulmonary disease: a pilot study. *J. Altern. Complement. Med.* Mar 2009;15(3):225-234.

103. Smeulders ES, van Haastregt JC, Ambergen T, Janssen-Boyne JJ, van Eijk JT, Kempen GI. The impact of a self-management group programme on health behaviour and healthcare utilization among congestive heart failure patients. *Eur J Heart Fail.* Jun 2009;11(6):609-616.

104. Andryukhin A, Frolova E, Vaes B, Degryse J. The impact of a nurse-led care programme on events and physical and psychosocial parameters in patients with heart failure with preserved ejection fraction: a randomized clinical trial in primary care in Russia. *Eur J Gen Pract.* Dec 2010;16(4):205-214.

105. Burke V, Mansour J, Beilin LJ, Mori TA. Long-term follow-up of participants in a health promotion program for treated hypertensives (ADAPT). *Nutr Metab Cardiovasc Dis.* Mar 2008;18(3):198-206.

106. Pierce JP, Watson DS, Knights S, Gliddon T, Williams S, Watson R. A controlled trial of health education in the physician's office. *Prev. Med.* Mar 1984;13(2):185-194.

107. Arnold CM. *Fall risk in older adults with hip osteoarthritis: Decreasing risk through education and aquatic exercise*, University of Saskatchewan (Canada); 2008.

APPENDIX A. SEARCH STRATEGY

PubMed Searched on February 13, 2012

Set# (concept)	Search Strategy	Results
#1 (things being done)	((("Health Education"[Mesh]) OR "Self Care"[Mesh]) OR lifestyle[Title/Abstract] OR counseling[Title/Abstract] OR "self[Title/Abstract] AND management"[Title/Abstract] OR "health[Title/Abstract] AND coaching"[Title/Abstract] OR "motivational[Title/Abstract] AND interviewing"[Title/Abstract] OR diet[Title/Abstract]))	393676
#2 (diseases of interest)	(hypertension[Title/Abstract] OR htn[Title/Abstract] OR chf[Title/Abstract] OR congestive[Title/Abstract] AND heart[Title/Abstract] AND failure[Title/Abstract] OR copd[Title/Abstract] OR chronic[Title/Abstract] AND obstructive[Title/Abstract] AND pulmonary[Title/Abstract] AND disease[Title/Abstract] OR arthritis[Title/Abstract] OR pain[Title/Abstract] AND management[Title/Abstract] OR fall[Title/Abstract] AND risk[Title/Abstract]) OR ((((("Hypertension"[Mesh] OR "Heart Failure"[Mesh] OR "Pulmonary Disease, Chronic Obstructive"[Mesh]) OR "Arthritis"[Mesh]) OR "Pain Management"[Mesh]) OR "Accidental Falls"[Mesh])) OR asthma OR "diabetes mellitus" [MeSH Terms] OR "diabetes"[Tiab]	615989
#3 (group aspect)	(((group[Title] OR groups[Title] OR share[Title] OR shared[Title]) OR ("Self-Help Groups"[Mesh])) NOT (("shared decision making") OR ("focus group") OR ("food group")))	163027
#4 (group aspect phrases)	"group education" OR "group attention control" OR "group sessions" OR "group therapy" OR "education group" OR "group program" OR "group programme" OR "group programs" OR "group programmes" OR "group interventions" OR "group exercise" OR "small group" OR "group strategy" OR "group relaxation" OR "group teaching" OR "group work" OR "group learning" OR "multidisciplinary intervention" OR "interdisciplinary intervention" OR "group session" OR "group patient visit" OR "nurse-led shared care" OR "nurse facilitated group" OR "group clinic" OR "group based self management" OR "peer led self management" OR "group or usual care" OR "group care" OR "peer led"	46864
#5 (false phrases)	"age group" OR "study group" OR "research group" OR "working group" OR "group practice" OR "group home" OR "youth group" OR "group foster home"	163923
#6 (group visits inclusive)	#3 OR #4	203980
#7	#6 AND #2 AND #1	1133
#8	#7 NOT #5	979
After deduplication from previous search		817

CINAHL (EBSCO) searched Monday, February 13, 2012 4:18:16 PM

Concept	Search Strategy	Results
Things being done	S8 S1 or S2 or S3 or S4 or S5 or S6 or S7 144186 S7 (MH "Diet+") 49615 S6 (MH "Motivational Interviewing") 758 S5 "health coaching" 68 S4 "self management" 4061 S3 (MH "Peer Counseling") OR "lifestyle counseling" 618 S2 (MH "Self Care+") 23157 S1 (MH "Health Education+") 77695	144186
Diseases of interest	S18 S9 or S10 or S11 or S12 or S13 or S14 or S15 or S16 or S17 125262 S17 (MH "Accidental Falls") OR "accidental falls" 10196 S16 "pain management" 6993 S15 (MH "Arthritis") OR "arthritis" 21888 S14 (MH "Pulmonary Disease, Chronic Obstructive+") OR "copd" 8106 S13 (MH "Heart Failure+") OR "congestive heart failure" 19227 S12 "chf" 1736 S11 "htn" 153 S10 (MH "Hypertension") OR "hypertension" 41268 S9 (MH "Asthma+") OR "asthma" OR (MH"Diabetes+") OR "diabetes" 22332	125262
Group	S44 S19 or S21 or S23 or S24 or S25 or S26 or S27 or S28 or S29 or S30 or S31 or S32 or S33 or S34 or S35 or S36 or S37 or S38 or S39 or S40 or S41 or S42 or S43 11958 S43 "group care" 103 S42 "group or usual care" 107 S41 "peer led self management" 7 S40 "group based self management" 5 S39 "group clinic" 12 S38 "nurse-led shared care" 7 S37 "group patient visits" 2 S36 "interdisciplinary intervention" 32 S35 "multidisciplinary intervention" 82 S34 "group learning" 167 S33 "group work" 701 S32 "group teaching" 114 S31 "group relaxation" 6 S30 "group strategy" 13 S29 "small group" 1763 S28 "group exercise" 692 S27 "group intervention" 794 S26 "group programme" 105 S25 "group program" 165 S24 "education group" 231 S23 "group therapy" 889 S22 ""group sessions" 0 S21 "group attention control" 2 S20 ""group education"" 0 S19 (MH "Group Exercise") OR (MH "Support Groups+") 7180	11958

Concept	Search Strategy	Results
False Phrases	S55 S45 or S46 or S47 or S48 or S49 or S50 or S51 or S52 or S53 or S54 20032 S54 "group foster home" 0 S53 "youth group" 14 S52 "group home" 142 S51 "group practice" 1642 S50 "working group" 1276 S49 "research group" 597 S48 "study group" 4509 S47 "food group" 180 S46 "focus group" 5757 S45 "age group" 6066	20032
	S8 and S18 and S44 128	128
	S57 S56 NOT S55 **123**	123
After deduplication from previous searches		90

Database: PsycINFO <1806 to February Week 1 2012>

Concept	Search Strategy
Things being done	1 exp Health Education/ (12448) 2 exp Self Management/ or exp Health Promotion/ or exp Disease Management/ (17441) 3 exp Lifestyle/ or lifestyle counseling.mp. (6652) 4 health coaching.mp. (37) 5 exp Motivational Interviewing/ (800) 6 1 or 2 or 3 or 4 or 5 (35296)
Diseases of interest	7 asthma.mp. or exp Asthma/ (5016) 8 exp Hypertension/ or hypertention.mp. (4665) 9 exp Heart Disorders/ or congestive heart failure.mp. (9041) 10 copd.mp. or exp Chronic Obstructive Pulmonary Disease/ (951) 11 exp Rheumatoid Arthritis/ or exp Arthritis/ or arthritis.mp. or exp diabetes mellitus/ or diabetes.mp. (4170) 12 pain management.mp. or exp Pain Management/ (7290) 13 exp Falls/ or accidental falls.mp. (1089)

Concept	Search Strategy
Group	15 exp Group Discussion/ or exp Group Counseling/ (7568) 16 "group education".mp. (252) 17 "group attention control".mp. (2) 18 "group sessions".mp. (1970) 19 "group therapy".mp. (10895) 20 "education group".mp. (419) 21 "group programme".mp. (109) 22 "group program".mp. (703) 23 "group intervention".mp. (1995) 24 "group exercise".mp. (164) 25 "small group".mp. (6780) 26 "group strategy".mp. (42) 27 "group relaxation".mp. (55) 28 "group teaching".mp. (174) 29 "group work".mp. (3647) 30 "group learning".mp. (698) 31 "multidisciplinary intervention".mp. (104) 32 "interdisciplinary intervention".mp. (46) 33 "group session".mp. (492) 34 "group patient visits".mp. (3) 35 "nurse-led shared care".mp. (3) 36 "group clinic".mp. (14) 37 "group based self-management".mp. (3) 38 "peer led self management".mp. (6) 39 "group or usual care".mp. (5) 40 "group or usual care".mp. (5) 41 "group care".mp. (414) 42 "peer led".mp. (356) 43 15 or 16 or 17 or 18 or 19 or 20 or 21 or 22 or 23 or 24 or 25 or 26 or 27 or 28 or 29 or 30 or 31 or 32 or 33 or 34 or 35 or 36 or 37 or 38 or 39 or 40 or 41 or 42 (32430)
False Phrases	44 "study group".mp. (2935) 45 "age group".mp. (8248) 46 "research group".mp. (1167) 47 "working group".mp. (897) 48 "group practice".mp. (456) 49 "group home".mp. (782) 50 "youth group".mp. (122) 51 "group foster home".mp. (8) 52 44 or 45 or 46 or 47 or 48 or 49 or 50 or 51 (14552)
	53 6 and 14 and 43 (55)
	54 53 not 52 (55)
Deduplication	N=44 unique

Database: EBM Reviews - Cochrane Central Register of Controlled Trials <January 2012>

Concept	Search Strategy
Things being done	1 exp Health Education/ (7370) 2 exp Self Management/ or exp Health Promotion/ or exp Disease Management/ (5010) 3 exp Lifestyle/ or lifestyle counseling.mp. (1877) 4 health coaching.mp. (12) 5 exp Motivational Interviewing/ (0) 6 1 or 2 or 3 or 4 or 5 (12310)
Disease of interest	7 asthma.mp. or exp Asthma/ (18081) 8 exp Hypertension/ or hypertention.mp. (12184) 9 exp Heart Disorders/ or congestive heart failure.mp. (2610) 10 copd.mp. or exp Chronic Obstructive Pulmonary Disease/ (5428) 11 exp Rheumatoid Arthritis/ or exp Arthritis/ or arthritis.mp. or exp diabetes mellitus or diabetes.exp(8528) 12 pain management.mp. or exp Pain Management/ (1220) 13 exp Falls/ or accidental falls.mp. (617) 14 7 or 8 or 9 or 10 or 11 or 12 or 13 (47973)
Group	15 exp Group Discussion/ or exp Group Counseling/ (0) 16 "group education".mp. (203) 17 "group attention control".mp. (15) 18 "group sessions".mp. (445) 19 "group therapy".mp. (905) 20 "education group".mp. (289) 21 "group programme".mp. (70) 22 "group program".mp. (188) 23 "group intervention".mp. (1350) 24 "group exercise".mp. (428) 25 "small group".mp. (662) 26 "group strategy".mp. (8) 27 "group relaxation".mp. (40) 28 "group teaching".mp. (42) 29 "group work".mp. (65) 30 "group learning".mp. (42) 31 "multidisciplinary intervention".mp. (50) 32 "interdisciplinary intervention".mp. (18) 33 "group session".mp. (85) 34 "group patient visits".mp. (1) 35 "nurse-led shared care".mp. (3) 36 "group clinic".mp. (27) 37 "group based self-management".mp. (4) 38 "peer led self management".mp. (1) 39 "group or usual care".mp. (156) 40 "group or usual care".mp. (156) 41 "group care".mp. (50) 42 "peer led".mp. (128) 43 15 or 16 or 17 or 18 or 19 or 20 or 21 or 22 or 23 or 24 or 25 or 26 or 27 or 28 or 29 or 30 or 31 or 32 or 33 or 34 or 35 or 36 or 37 or 38 or 39 or 40 or 41 or 42 (4846)

Concept	Search Strategy
False phrases	44 "study group".mp. (10409) 45 "age group".mp. (1455) 46 "research group".mp. (752) 47 "working group".mp. (210) 48 "group practice".mp. (165) 49 "group home".mp. (82) 50 "youth group".mp. (5) 51 "group foster home".mp. (0) 52 44 or 45 or 46 or 47 or 48 or 49 or 50 or 51 (12995)
	53 6 and 14 and 43 (175) 54 53 not 52 (167)

APPENDIX B. INCLUSION AND EXCLUSION CRITERIA

This criteria is for use in screening full-text articles to address the following key questions:

KQ1. In adults with chronic medical conditions, how do group visits compared to usual care affect the following:

(1) medication adherence, biophysical markers [laboratory markers of health states (e.g., HbA1c) or physiological measures (e.g., blood pressure)]
(2) symptom status, functional status, disease-specific or all-cause mortality, patient satisfaction
(3) utilization of medical resources, health care costs
(4) adverse outcomes (e.g., patient confidentiality, participation/missed appointments)?

KQ2. For adults with chronic medical conditions, do the effects of group visits vary by patient characteristics? Characteristics of interest include medical diagnosis, severity of disease, and comorbidities.

KQ3. (Depending on the size and comparability of elements identified in the literature) Which components of group visits are associated with greater intervention effects?

---

1. Is the full text of the article in English?
    Yes..Proceed to #2
    No..Code **X1**. STOP

2. Is the article a primary study that presents findings based on original data collection; or a systematic review of primary studies?
    Yes..Proceed to #3
    No..Code **X2**. Go to #6

3. Does the study population include adults with chronic medical conditions, specifically DM, HTN, CHF, COPD, asthma, arthritis, pain management, or history of falls?
    Yes..Proceed to #4
    No..Code **X3**. Go to #6

4. Does the study evaluate the effects of an intervention consisting of group visits led by non-prescribing facilitators (e.g., dietitians, nurses, social workers, peer educators, psychologists, pulmonary technicians, physical therapists)? Group visits may include prescribing practitioners (e.g., pharmacists, nurse practitioners, physician assistants, physicians) if they function in an advisory capacity only and do not provide individual care plans or medication management.
    Yes..Proceed to #5
    No, not a group visit intervention ....Code **X4**. Go to #6
    No, a group visit that includes individualized treatment by a prescribing provider..Code **X4-SMA**
    No, a group visit in the diabetes mellitus clinical area that was published prior to the 1998 UKPDS study...Code **X4-pre UKPDS**

5. Is the study design one of the following:
   An RCT or a systematic review/meta-analysis that includes RCTs..........................Code **I**
   An observational/quasi-experimental study.. Code **O**
   None of the above ....Code **X5**. Proceed to #6

6. Is the article potentially useful for background, discussion, or reference-mining?
   Yes.. Add code **B**. STOP
   No... STOP

Codes to use for abstract screening:

X = Exclude
B = Background
I = Include
O = Observational quasi/experimental study
SMA = Not relevant for Group Visits but may be useful for review of Shared Medical Appointments

PICOTS

Patients – Patients with DM, HTN, CHF, COPD, asthma, arthritis, pain management, history of falls.

Exclude comorbid serious mental illness such as schizophrenia. Studies with patients who have comorbid depression may be included.

Intervention – Group visits led by individuals who are non-prescribing health professionals and lay facilitators (e.g., dietitians, nurses, social workers, peer educators, psychologists, pulmonary technicians, physical therapists). Group visits may include prescribing providers (e.g., physicians, pharmacists, advanced practice nurses, physician assistants) if they function in an advisory capacity only (i.e., do not provide individual care plans or medication management).

Exclude the following:
- support groups with no education component
- multicomponent interventions for which a group visit is an optional but not required element
- multicomponent interventions that contain a required group visit but the independent effects of the group visit component cannot be evaluated separately
- interventions that focus on completion of established exercise or relaxation modalities (e.g. yoga, tai chi, meditation classes) with no education component. However, a group visit that teaches and/or demonstrates tailored exercises would be included.

Comparator – Usual care, non-group visit care

Outcome – Biophysical markers (HbA1c, lipids); physiological measures (BP); control of these markers/measures; rehospitalizations; medication adherence; ED visits; functional status; patient satisfaction; patient participation; attrition rates; utilization of medical resources, health care costs; and adverse outcomes.

Timing – To be determined. We may want to allow for sufficiently long group visit interventions to observe differences between groups

Setting – Any

APPENDIX C. QUALITY ASSESSMENT

Definition of "good," "fair," and "poor" designations

Studies rated "good" have the least risk of bias, and results are considered valid. Good-quality studies include clear descriptions of the population, setting, interventions, and comparison groups; a valid method for allocation of patients to treatment; low dropout rates and clear reporting of dropouts; appropriate means for preventing bias; and appropriate measurement of outcomes.

Studies rated "fair" are susceptible to some bias, but it is not sufficient to invalidate results. These studies do not meet all the criteria for a "good" quality rating, but there is no indication that study flaws are likely to cause major bias. The study may be missing information, making it difficult to assess limitations and potential problems. The "fair" quality category is broad, and studies in this category can vary in their strengths and limitations. The results from fair studies range from valid to probably valid.

Studies rated "poor" have substantial flaws that imply biases in various rated categories that may invalidate results. They have a serious or "fatal" flaw in design, analysis, or reporting, including: large amounts of missing information, discrepancies in reporting, or raise serious concerns about the delivery of the intervention. The results of these studies are as likely to reflect flaws in the study design as they are to reflect true differences between compared groups. We did not exclude studies rated poor quality a priori, but poor quality studies were considered to be less valid than higher-quality studies when synthesizing the evidence, particularly when discrepancies between studies were present.

Group Visits Focusing on Education for the Management of Chronic Conditions in Adults

Appendix Table C1. Quality assessment and methodological characteristics of individual studies in randomized controlled trials of group visits

Study	Selection: random sequence	Selection: allocation concealment	Blinding: participants	Blinding: personnel	Detection: assessors blinded	Attrition: address missing	Reporting: no selective reporting	Participation (% enrolled among eligible individuals)	Attrition (% loss to followup among N randomized)	Study quality (Good/Fair/Poor)
Abdulwadud, 1999[49]	Unclear	Unclear	No	No	Unclear	Unclear	Unclear	71	38	Poor
Ackerman, 2012[31]	Yes	Yes	No	No	No	Yes	Yes	25	22	Fair
Adolfsson, 2007[75]	Unclear	Yes	Unclear	Unclear	Unclear	Yes	Yes	53	13	Fair
Allen, 1995[50]	Unclear	Unclear	Unclear	No	Unclear	Yes	Unclear	NA*	3	Poor
Anderson, 2005[76]	Unclear	Unclear	Unclear	Unclear	Unclear	Yes	Yes	NA*	6	Poor
Arnold, 2010[45]	Yes	Yes	No	No	Yes	Yes	Yes	55	23	Fair
Baghianimoghadam, 2010[67]	Unclear	No	No	No	No	NR	Yes	NR	NR	Poor
Balcazar, 2009[64]	Yes	Unclear	No	No	Unclear	Yes	Yes	NR	0	Poor
Barlow, 2000[32]	Yes	Yes	Unclear	Unclear	Unclear	Yes	Yes	NR	22	Fair
Bestall, 2003[54]	Yes	Yes	Unclear	Unclear	Unclear	Yes	Yes	NR	16	Fair
Bolton, 1991[51]	Unclear	Unclear	Unclear	Unclear	Yes	Yes	Yes	45	7	Fair
Breedland, 2011[33]	Yes	Yes	No	No	Yes	Yes	Yes	NR	6	Good
Brown, 2002[15]	Unclear	Unclear	No	No	Unclear	No	No	NR	NR	Poor
Brown, 2005[16]	Unclear	Unclear	Unclear	Unclear	Unclear	Unclear	Yes	NR	NR	Poor
Buszewicz, 2006[34]	Yes	Yes	Unclear	Unclear	Unclear	Yes	Yes	30	24	Fair
Chang, 2005[59]	Yes	Unclear	No	No	No	Yes	Yes	17	13	Fair
Clemson, 2004[24]	Yes	Unclear	No	Unclear	Yes	Yes	Yes	NA*	15	Good
Deakin, 2006[71]	Yes	Yes	Yes	No	No	Yes	Yes	20	32	Fair
De Greef, 2011[73]	Yes	Yes	No	No	Yes	Yes	Yes	78	5	Good
Dejesus, 2009[77]	Unclear	Unclear	Unclear	Unclear	Unclear	No	Yes	13	55	Poor
Effing, 2011[55]	Yes	Unclear	No	No	Unclear	Yes	Yes	41	11	Fair
Elzen, 2007[89]	Unclear	Unclear	Unclear	Unclear	N/A	Yes	Yes	26	10	Poor
Ersek, 2003[97]	Unclear	Unclear	Unclear	No	Unclear	Yes	Yes	NA*	13	Fair
Ettinger, 1997[22]	Yes	Yes	Unclear	Unclear	Yes	Yes	Yes	53	17	Fair
Figar, 2006[65]	Yes	Yes	Unclear	Unclear	Yes	Yes	Yes	NR	17	Good
Freeman, 2002[36]	Unclear	Unclear	Unclear	Unclear	Yes	Unclear	Yes	94	23	Fair
Fu, 2003[90]	Yes	No	No	No	No	Yes	Yes	NA*	13	Fair

Group Visits Focusing on Education for the Management of Chronic Conditions in Adults — Evidence-based Synthesis Program

Study	Selection: random sequence	Selection: allocation concealment	Blinding: participants	Blinding: personnel	Detection: assessors blinded	Attrition: address missing	Reporting: no selective reporting	Participation (% enrolled among eligible individuals)	Attrition (% loss to followup among N randomized)	Study quality (Good/Fair/Poor)
Giraudet-Le Quintrec, 2007[37]	Yes	Yes	Unclear	Unclear	Yes	Unclear	Yes	18	9	Fair
Gustavsson, 2010[98]	Yes	Yes	No	Yes	Yes	Yes	Yes	84	20	Good
Hammond, 1999[23]	Unclear	Unclear	No	No	Yes	Yes	Yes	NR	31	Fair
Hammond, 2008[47]	Yes	Yes	No	No	Unclear	Yes	Yes	46	37	Fair
Haugli, 2000[28]	Unclear	Unclear	Unclear	Unclear	Unclear	Yes	Yes	NR	33	Poor
Haugli, 2003[95]	Unclear	Unclear	Unclear	Unclear	Unclear	Yes	Yes	NA*	30	Poor
Hewlett, 2011[38]	Yes	Yes	No	No	Yes	Yes	Yes	15	24	Good
Hornsten, 2008[17]	Unclear	Unclear	No	No	No	Yes	Yes	NR	14	Fair
Kaplan, 1981[39]	Unclear	Unclear	Unclear	Unclear	Yes	Yes	Yes	NR	35	Poor
Khunti, 2012[68]	Yes	Yes	Unclear	Unclear	Unclear	Yes	Yes	NA*	11	Good
Kulzer, 2007[72]	Unclear	Unclear	Unclear	Unclear	Unclear	Yes	Yes	50	6	Fair
Kunik, 2008[57]	Yes	Yes	No	No	Yes	Yes	Yes	19	55	Good
Lorig, 1985[40]	Unclear	Unclear	Unclear	Unclear	Unclear	Yes	Yes	NA*	16	Fair
Lorig, 1999[41]	Unclear	Unclear	Unclear	Unclear	Unclear	Yes	Yes	NR	17	Poor
Lorig, 2003[91]	Unclear	Unclear	Unclear	Unclear	Yes	Unclear	Yes	51	51	Fair
Lorig, 2004[29]	Yes	Yes	No	Yes	Yes	Yes	Yes	84	32	Good
Lorig, 2009[69]	Unclear	Unclear	No	No	Unclear	Yes	Yes	NA*	15	Fair
Lujan, 2007[78]	Unclear	Unclear	No	No	Yes	Yes	Yes	NR	6	Fair
Melkus, 2010[13]	Yes	Unclear	Unclear	Unclear	Unclear	Yes	Yes	NA*	11	Fair
Miller, 2002[79]	Yes	Unclear	No	No	Unclear	Yes	Yes	NA*	6	Fair
Moore, 2006[58]	Yes	Yes	No	No	No	Yes	Yes	50	19	Fair
Nessman, 1980[62]	Unclear	Unclear	No	No	Unclear	Yes	Yes	36	0	Poor
Ninot, 2011[56]	Yes	Yes	No	No	Yes	Yes	Yes	NA*	16	Good
Patel, 2009[35]	Yes	Yes	Unclear	Unclear	Unclear	Yes	Yes	30	24	Fair
Philis-Tsimikas, 2011[18]	Yes	Yes	No	No	Probably	No	Yes	NR	25	Poor
Raji, 2002[80]	Unclear	Unclear	Unclear	Unclear	Unclear	Unclear	Unclear	33	NR	Poor
Rickheim, 2002[74]	No	Unclear	Unclear	Unclear	Unclear	Unclear	Yes	NR	46	Poor
Riemsma, 2003[42]	Unclear	Unclear	Unclear	Unclear	Unclear	Yes	Yes	26	17	Fair

Group Visits Focusing on Education for the Management of Chronic Conditions in Adults

Evidence-based Synthesis Program

Study	Selection: random sequence	Selection: allocation concealment	Blinding: participants	Blinding: personnel	Detection: assessors blinded	Attrition: address missing	Reporting: no selective reporting	Participation (% enrolled among eligible individuals)	Attrition (% loss to followup among N randomized)	Study quality (Good/Fair/Poor)
Rosal, 2011[19]	Yes	Unclear	No	No	Yes	Unclear	Yes	57	16	Fair
Rujiwatthanakorn, 2011[63]	Yes	Yes	No	No	No	Yes	Yes	70	12	Poor
Ryan, 1996[46]	Unclear	Unclear	Unclear	Unclear	Unclear	Unclear	Yes	NR	NR	Poor
Rygg, 2012[21]	Yes	Yes	No	No	No	Unclear	Yes	91	9	Fair
Sarkadi, 2004[81]	Yes	Yes	No	No	No	Unclear	Yes	92	17	Fair
Scain, 2009[82]	Unclear	Unclear	No	No	No	Unclear	Yes	86	0	Fair
Scala, 2008[66]	Yes	Unclear	No	No	Unclear	No	Yes	NR	42	Poor
Schillinger, 2009[30]	Yes	Unclear	No	No	Unclear	Yes	Yes	73	10	Fair
Sevick, 2009[43]	Yes	Yes	No	No	Yes	Yes	Yes	NR	20	Good
Sharifirad, 2012[83]	Unclear	Unclear	Unclear	Unclear	Unclear	Unclear	Unclear	NR	3	Poor
Shumway-Cook, 2007[25]	Yes	Yes	Unclear	Unclear	Yes	Yes	Yes	88	5	Fair
Smeulders, 2010[60]	Yes	Yes	No	No	Yes	Yes	Yes	44	16	Good
Smeulders, 2010[27]	Yes	Yes	No	No	Yes	Yes	Yes	44	16	Good
Snyder, 1987[52]	Unclear	Unclear	No	No	Unclear	Unclear	Unclear	NR	5	Poor
Sperl-Hillen, 2011[84]	Unclear	Unclear	Unclear	Unclear	Unclear	Yes	Yes	82	2	Fair
Steed, 2005[85]	No	No	Unclear	Unclear	Unclear	Yes	Yes	51	16	Poor
Surwit, 2002[20]	Unclear	Unclear	Unclear	Unclear	Unclear	Unclear	Yes	NR	24	Poor
Svetkey, 2009[26]	Yes	Yes	No	Yes	Yes	Unclear	Unclear	56	12	Good
Taal, 1993[44]	Unclear	Unclear	Unclear	Unclear	Unclear	No	Yes	54	24	Poor
Toobert, 2011[86]	Yes	No	Unclear	Unclear	Yes	Yes	Yes	61	22	Fair
Vlaeyen, 1996[96]	Unclear	Unclear	Unclear	Unclear	Unclear	Yes	Yes	NR	20	Poor
Weinger, 2011[14]	Yes	Unclear	Unclear	Unclear	Unclear	Yes	Yes	89	3	Fair
Wilson, 1993[48]	Yes	Yes	No	Yes	Yes	No	Yes	56	14	Fair
Wilson, 2008[53]	Yes	Yes	No	No	Unclear	Unclear	Yes	60	NR	Fair
Zapotoczky, 2001[88]	Unclear	Unclear	Unclear	Unclear	Unclear	Unclear	Yes	100	0	Poor

Abbreviations: NA = not applicable; NR = not reported.
* Participation among all potentially eligible participants could not be calculated because subjects were recruited via community advertisement.

Table C2. Total number of outcome measures reported in studies of group visit interventions focusing on education for the management of chronic disease

Study	Clinical area	Category	Outcomes/Measures	Subscale	Total outcomes examined
Taal, 1993[44]	Arthritis	Anxiety/Depression	VAS	anxiety	20
				depression	
		Functional status or disability	DUTCH-AIMS, M-HAQ	disability	
				dexterity	
				household activities	
				physical activities	
		Health status	HbA1c (marker disease activity)	N/A	
		Pain	joint tenderness score (Richie et al. 1968)	N/A	
			VAS	arthritis impact	
				pain	
		Self-efficacy	activities (Lorig et al. 1989)	N/A	
			endurance (Lorig et al. 1989)	N/A	
			exercise (Lorig et al. 1989)	N/A	
			function (five-point scale)	N/A	
			other symptoms (five-point scale)	N/A	
			pain (Lorig et al. 1989)	N/A	
			relaxation (Lorig et al. (1989)	N/A	
			VAS	social activities	
		Biophysical	ESR	blood samples	
			thrombocytes	N/A	
Lorig, 2004[29]	Arthritis	Anxiety/Depression	CESD	N/A	8
		Functional status or disability	ALS (role function)	N/A	
			HAQ	disability	
		Pain	VAS	N/A	
		Quality of life	global severity arthritis	N/A	
		Self-efficacy	ASES	N/A	
		Utilization	total MD visits (last 6 mo)	N/A	
			total rheumatology visits (last 6 mo)	N/A	
Lorig, 1985[40]	Arthritis	Exercise tolerance	exercise (#/mo)	N/A	7
			relaxation (#/mo)	N/A	
		Functional status or disability	Stanford Health Assessment Questionnaire (0-3 scale) disability	N/A	
		Pain	pain (0-3 scale)		
			VAS	N/A	
		Self-efficacy	knowledge (0-10 scale)	N/A	
		Utilization	total MD visits (last 4 mo)	N/A	
Kaplan, 1981[39]	Arthritis	Psychometric	Human service scale 1	N/A	4
			Tennessee self-concept scale 1	N/A	
		Self-efficacy	knowledge	N/A	
		Anxiety/Depression	depression	N/A	

Study	Clinical area	Category	Outcomes/Measures	Subscale	Total outcomes examined
Hewlett, 2011[38]	Arthritis	Pain	VAS	pain	13
		Quality of life	RAQol	quality of life	
		Self-efficacy	AHI	N/A	
			RASE	N/A	
			VAS	coping	
		Anxiety/Depression	HADS	anxiety	
				depression	
		Disease severity	VAS	disease activity	
		Fatigue	MAF	fatigue impact	
			VAS	fatigue impact	
		Functional status or disability	HAQ	disability	
			PIHAQ	impact disability	
			VAS	severity	
Hammond, 2008[47]	Arthritis	Anxiety/Depression	HAQ	anxiety	21
				psychological distress	
				depression	
		Exercise tolerance	self-management exercise	N/A	
		Fatigue	VAS	fatigue	
		Functional status or disability	early morning stiffness	N/A	
			HAQ	functional ability	
		Pain	VAS	pain	
		Self-efficacy	cognitive symptom management	N/A	
			AHI	helplessness	
				perceived control	
			ASCQ	action	
				contemplation	
				maintenance	
				pre-contemplation	
			ASES	Pain + other symptoms	
			perceived health (scale (0-100))	N/A	
			RASE	N/A	
		Self-efficacy/ Functional status	fatigue management (scale 1-6)	N/A	
			joint protection (scale 1-6)	N/A	
		Utilization	total MD visits (last 6-12 mo)	N/A	
Breedland, 2011[33]	Arthritis	Exercise tolerance	physical performance	aerobic capacity	8
				muscle strength LE	
				muscle strength UE	
		Health status	Dutch-AIMS2 – health status	physical health	
				psychological health	
				social interaction	
		Self-efficacy/ Functional status and disability/pain	ASES – self efficacy	function	
				pain + other symptoms	

Study	Clinical area	Category	Outcomes/Measures	Subscale	Total outcomes examined
Riemsma, 2003[42]	Arthritis	Disease severity	DAS28 (disease activity)	N/A	20
		Exercise tolerance	health behavior (7 items on 5-point scale)	endurance exercises	
				physical exercises	
				relaxation exercises	
				self-management	
		Fatigue	VAS (fatigue)	N/A	
		Functional status or disability/pain	AIMS2	physical function	
				pain	
		Pain/Self-efficacy	CORS	coping with pain	
		Quality of life	AIMS2	health status: affect	
		Self-efficacy	social interactions (Revenson)	emotional support	
				esteem support	
				informational support	
				overprotection	
				problematic support	
				tangible support	
			CORS	coping with limitations	
		Self-efficacy/ Functional status and disability/ Pain	SES	self-efficacy	
				other symptoms (depression, fatigue, frustration)	
				self-efficacy function	
				self-efficacy pain	
Giraudet-Le Quintrec, 2007[37]	Arthritis	Anxiety/Depression	HADS	anxiety	16
				depression	
		Disease severity	DAS28 (disease activity)	N/A	
		Exercise tolerance	Baecke questionnaire	physical activity	
		Fatigue	FACIT-F	N/A	
		Knowledge	rheumatoid arthritis knowledge (10-item)	N/A	
		Patient satisfaction	satisfaction with the program (Likert scale)	N/A	
		Quality of life	EMIR (AIMS2)	physical	
				psychological	
				social	
				symptomatic	
				work	
			HAQ	quality of life: unweighted	
				quality of life: with weighting	
		Self-efficacy	AHI (coping)	N/A	
		Utilization	EURIDISS	drug compliance	
Sevick, 2009[43]	Arthritis	Biophysical	BMI	N/A	7
		Functional status, pain, disability	WOMAC	degree of difficulty	
				function	
				stiffness	
				pain	
		Physical performance	6MWT	N/A	
			stair climb	N/A	

Study	Clinical area	Category	Outcomes/Measures	Subscale	Total outcomes examined
Barlow, 2000[32]	Arthritis	Anxiety/Depression	HADS	anxiety	12
				depression	
			HADS, PANAS	psychologic well-being	
		Fatigue; pain	VAS	fatigue	
				pain	
		Pain/Self-efficacy	ASE	pain	
		Quality of life	PANAS	negative affect	
				positive affect	
		Self-efficacy	ASE	other symptoms	
			HAQ (dietary habit)	N/A	
		Utilization	communication with physician	N/A	
Buszewicz, 2006[34]	Arthritis	Pain	ASE	other	8
				pain	
			WOMAC	pain	
		Quality of life	SF-36	mental health	
		Functional status or disability	WOMAC	physical function	
				stiffness	
		Quality of life	SF-36	physical health	
		Anxiety/Depression	HADS	anxiety	
				depression	
Freeman, 2002[36]	Arthritis	Functional status or disability	28 JC	N/A	12
			EMS	N/A	
		Pain	ESR (duration of early morning stiffness)	N/A	
			VAS	N/A	
		Quality of life	AIMS2	affect	
				current health	
				physical functional ability	
				symptoms	
		Self-efficacy	ASES	N/A	
			RAI	helplessness	
				internality	
			TSES	N/A	
Ettinger, 1997[22]	Arthritis	Exercise tolerance	aerobic capacity (0-3 Likert scale)	N/A	10
			aerobic training	N/A	
			knee pain (1-6 Likert scale)	N/A	
			physical performance	endurance	
				distance (6MWT)	
				mobility	
				strength	
			resistance training	N/A	
		Functional status or disability	self-reported disability (FAST, Likert scale)	N/A	
		Utilization	x-ray	N/A	

Study	Clinical area	Category	Outcomes/Measures	Subscale	Total outcomes examined
Hammond, 1999[23]	Arthritis	Functional status or disability	HAQ	functional ability	11
			HJAM (range of movement and joint deformity)	N/A	
		Pain	HAQ	hand pain	
			HJC (number of painful/tender hand joints)	N/A	
			VAS (hand pain)	N/A	
		Physical performance	grip strength	N/A	
		Self-efficacy	AHI	N/A	
			ASES	N/A	
			JP (self-reported homework)	N/A	
			JPBA (joint protection behavior)	N/A	
			JPKA (knowledge)	N/A	
Lorig, 1999[41]	Arthritis	Anxiety/Depression	CESD	depression	9
		Exercise tolerance	aerobic exercise	N/A	
			range of motion exercise	N/A	
		Functional status or disability	HAQ	disability	
		Pain	VNS (modified VAS)	pain	
		Quality of life	MOS	general health/self-rated health	
		Self-efficacy	HAQ	self-efficacy	
		Utilization	MD visits (last 6 mo)	N/A	
			medication use (NSAIDs)	N/A	
Patel, 2009[35]	Arthritis	Costs	VAS	costs to patient, family, friends	11
				indirect costs	
				social care costs	
				total costs, societal perspective	
				total health costs	
		Pain	EQ-5D: VAS	utility index	
		Quality of life	EuroQol: VAS	quality of life	
			QALYs	quality adjusted life years	
			SF-36	mental health	
				physical health	
				cost effective on basis of QoL	

Study	Clinical area	Category	Outcomes/Measures	Subscale	Total outcomes examined
Ackerman, 2012[31]	Arthritis	Pain	WOMAC	pain	15
		Quality of life	AQoL	arthritis related quality of life	
			heiQ	acquisition	
				activity	
				attitudes/approaches	
				emotional distress	
				engagement	
				health service navigation	
				self-monitoring	
				social integration/ support	
			HRQOL	health related quality of life	
		Health status	MAPT (arthritis disease severity)	N/A	
		Functional status or disability	WOMAC	physical function	
				stiffness	
		Anxiety/Depression	K10 (distress)	N/A	
Wilson, 1993[48]	Asthma	Exercise tolerance	change in ph. activity (1 year)	N/A	8
		Health status	# symptomatic days (1 year)	N/A	
			asthma status (5 mo)	N/A	
			relative "bother" (1 year)	N/A	
		Self-management	improved MDI technique (1 year)	N/A	
			improvements bedr. environment (1 year)	N/A	
		Utilization	acute visit rates	N/A	
			difference in acute visit rates	N/A	
Abdulwadud, 1999[49]	Asthma	Quality of life	AQLQ	breathlessness	7
				concern for health	
				mood disturbance	
				social disruption	
		Self-efficacy	AGKQ	knowledge	
			HAAS	self-mgmt: rapid onset	
				self-mgmt: slow onset	
Allen, 1995[50]	Asthma	Biophysical	FEV/FVC	adequacy of medical treatment	4
				morbidity	
		Self-management	compliance with meds	N/A	
		Self-efficacy	knowledge	N/A	
Bolton, 1991[51]	Asthma	Functional status or disability	days of limited activity	N/A	4
		Utilization	emergency room visits	N/A	
			hospitalization	N/A	
			physician visits	N/A	
Kritikos, 2007[101]	Asthma	Disease Severity	asthma severity	N/A	6
		Quality of life	AQLQ	total quality of life	
		Self-management	MARS	medication adherence	
		Self-efficacy	CQ	knowledge	
			optimal DPI	N/A	
			optimal MDI	N/A	

Study	Clinical area	Category	Outcomes/Measures	Subscale	Total outcomes examined
Snyder, 1987[52]	Asthma	Disease severity	symptom severity	N/A	4
		Self-efficacy	ASES	self-efficacy	
			attitudes about asthma (AASA 24-item)	N/A	
			BIQ (knowledge)		
Wilson, 2008[53]	COPD	Quality of life	MRC (dyspnea)	N/A	4
		Self-efficacy	abstinence from smoking validation, self-report (IC)	N/A	
			HSI (addiction)	N/A	
			stages of change (5 categories: pre-contemplation, contemplation, preparation, action, ex-smoker)	N/A	
Kunik, 2008[57]	COPD	Exercise tolerance	6MWT	N/A	18
		Quality of life	BAI	anxiety	
			BDI-II	depressive symptoms	
			CRQ	Qol: fatigue	
				Qol: mastery	
				Qol: dyspnoea	
				Qol: emotion	
			SF-36	emotional composite	
				general health	
				mental health	
				pain	
				physical composite	
				physical function	
				role-emotionally	
				role-physical	
				social function	
				vitality	
		Utilization	use of health services	N/A	
Bestall, 2003[54]	COPD	Anxiety/Depression	HADS	anxiety	12
				depression	
		Exercise tolerance	shuttle walking		
			walking distance		
		Quality of life	CRDQ (7-pt Likert scale)	emotional function	
				fatigue	
				mastery	
				dyspnoea	
			SGRQ	health status: activity	
				health status: impacts	
				health status: symptoms	
		Self-efficacy	EADL	N/A	

Study	Clinical area	Category	Outcomes/Measures	Subscale	Total outcomes examined
Donesky-Cuenco, 2009[102]	COPD	Biophysical	FEVI/FVC	N/A	16
		Quality of life	SF-36	mental component	
				physical component	
		Quality of life/ Functional status or disability	FPI total	functional performance	
		Self-efficacy	CRQ	mastery	
		Anxiety	SSAI	N/A	
		Anxiety/Depression	CESD	N/A	
		Exercise tolerance	incremental cycle (ergometry)	N/A	
			hamstring flex tq/bw 180	N/A	
			hamstring flexion tq/bw 90	N/A	
			quads extension tq/bw 180	N/A	
			quads extension tq/bw 90	N/A	
		Fatigue	CRQ	fatigue	
		Quality of life	CRQ	emotional	
			CRQ (Borg) dyspnea	N/A	
			FEVI (lung function)	N/A	
Effing, 2011[55]	COPD	Anxiety/Depression	HADS	anxiety	14
				depression	
		Biophysical	FFM	N/A	
		Exercise tolerance	CRQ	dyspnoea	
			ESWT	distance	
			ISWT	distance	
			max exercise capacity	N/A	
			steps per day (pedometer)	N/A	
		Fatigue	CRQ	fatigue	
		Quality of life	CCQ	functional state	
				mental state	
				symptoms	
				emotional function	
		Self-efficacy	CRQ	mastery	
Ninot, 2011[56]	COPD	Exercise tolerance	6MWD	N/A	16
			daily physical activity (Voorrips)	N/A	
		Quality of life	HRQoL	N/A	
			SGRQ	health status: impacts	
				health status: symptoms	
				health status: total	
				health status: activity	
			utilization	N/A	
			VAS	dyspnea	
			NHP	physical mobility	
			pulmonary function	N/A	
		Quality of life/Pain	NHP	pain	
				sleep	
				energy	
				social isolation	
				emotional reaction	

Study	Clinical area	Category	Outcomes/Measures	Subscale	Total outcomes examined
Fu, 2003[90]	COPD, multiple morbidity	Fatigue	fatigue	N/A	13
		Functional status or disability	disability	N/A	
		Health behavior	aerobic exercise	N/A	
		Health status	depression	N/A	
			health distress	N/A	
			pain	N/A	
			self-rated health	N/A	
			shortness of breath	N/A	
			social and role activity limitations	N/A	
		Self-management	cognitive symptom management	N/A	
		Self-efficacy	Self-efficacy in self-management	managing symptoms	
				managing disease in general	
		Utilization	hospital stays	N/A	
Dejesus, 2009[77]	Diabetes	Biophysical	DBP	N/A	3
			SBP	N/A	
		Utilization	# of MD and RN visits	N/A	
Elzen, 2007[89]	Diabetes, multiple morbidity	Exercise tolerance	self-management behavior: frequency of exercise	N/A	12
		Quality of life	RAND-36	general health	
				physical functioning	
				role limitations (physical problem)	
				physical component: pain	
				mental health	
				role limitations (emotional problem)	
				social functioning	
				vitality	
		Self-efficacy	GSES-16	self-efficacy	
			self-management behavior: cognitive symptom mgmt	N/A	
		Utilization	communication with physician	N/A	
Lorig, 2003[91]	Diabetes, multiple morbidity	Anxiety/Depression	health status: health distress	N/A	13
		Exercise tolerance	behavior: exercise (total min per week)	N/A	
		Fatigue	health status: fatigue	N/A	
		Functional status or disability	health status: role function	N/A	
		Health status	health status: self-reported health	N/A	
		Pain	health status: pain?	N/A	
		Self-efficacy	behavior: current use tobacco	N/A	
			behavior: mental stress mgmt	N/A	
			self-efficacy (4-item scale)	N/A	
		Utilization	communication with physician (4-item scale)	N/A	
			ER visits	N/A	
			hospital days	N/A	
			physician visits	N/A	

Study	Clinical area	Category	Outcomes/Measures	Subscale	Total outcomes examined
Weinger, 2011[14]	Diabetes	Anxiety/Depression	Depression (Brief Symptom Inventory-18)	N/A	12
			diabetes-related distress (5-point Likert scale)	N/A	
		Biophysical	BMI	N/A	
			HbA1c	N/A	
			HDL cholesterol	N/A	
			LDL cholesterol	N/A	
		Exercise tolerance	mean 3-day pedometer	N/A	
		Quality of life	diabetes (100-point scale)	N/A	
		Self-management	glucose meter checks	N/A	
		Self-efficacy	controlled coping styles	N/A	
			self-care inventory (5-point Likert scale)	N/A	
			self-efficacy (5-point Likert scale)	N/A	
Khunti, 2012[68]	Diabetes	Anxiety/Depression	HADS	N/A	27
		Biophysical	blood pressure	N/A	
			BMI	N/A	
			diastolic BP	N/A	
			HbA1c	N/A	
			HDL cholesterol	N/A	
			LDL cholesterol	N/A	
			systolic BP	N/A	
			total cholesterol	N/A	
			triglycerides	N/A	
			UKPDS 10 yr CHD risk	N/A	
			Waist circumference	N/A	
		Health behavior	physical activity	N/A	
			smoking status	N/A	
		Health status	Problem areas in diabetes questionnaire (emotional distress)	N/A	
		Quality of life	WHO QOL-BREF	main scale	
				health satisfaction	
				physical QOL	
				psychological QOL	
				social QOL	
				environmental QOL	
		Self-efficacy	IPQ-R	perceived knowledge (coherence)	
				perceived illness duration (timeline)	
				perceived self control	
				perceived seriousness	
				perceived impact	

Study	Clinical area	Category	Outcomes/Measures	Subscale	Total outcomes examined
Adolfsson, 2007[75]	Diabetes	Biophysical	BMI	N/A	6
			HbA1c	N/A	
			weight	N/A	
		Knowledge	VAS scale (confidence in DM knowledge)	N/A	
		Quality of life	Satisfaction with daily life (adapted WHO QOL)	N/A	
		Self-efficacy	10-item questionnaire	N/A	
Anderson, 2005[76]	Diabetes	Attitudes	seriousness of diabetes (Diabetes Attitude Scale-3)	N/A	10
		Biophysical	diastolic BP	N/A	
			HbA1c	N/A	
			serum cholesterol	N/A	
			systolic BP	N/A	
			weight	N/A	
		Knowledge	perceived understanding of diabetes	N/A	
		Self-efficacy	DES-SF (psychosocial self-efficacy)	N/A	
		Social and psychological factors	Diabetes Care Profile (DCP)	negative attitude	
				positive attitude	
Brown, 2005[16]	Diabetes	Biophysical	FBG (fasting blood glucose)	N/A	3
			HbA1c	N/A	
		Knowledge	diabetes knowledge	N/A	
Brown, 2002[15]	Diabetes	Biophysical	BMI	N/A	13
			cholesterol	N/A	
			FBG	N/A	
			HbA1c	N/A	
			height	N/A	
			triglycerides	N/A	
			weight	N/A	
		Knowledge	diabetes knowledge	N/A	
		Self-efficacy	health beliefs: barriers	N/A	
			health beliefs: benefits	N/A	
			health beliefs: control	N/A	
			health beliefs: impact of job	N/A	
			health beliefs: social support	N/A	
Davies, 2008[70]	Diabetes	Biophysical	BMI	N/A	11
			DBP	N/A	
			HbA1c	N/A	
			HDL	N/A	
			LDL	N/A	
			SBP	N/A	
			total cholesterol	N/A	
			triglycerides	N/A	
			waist circumference	N/A	
		Health behavior	physical activity	N/A	
			smoking status	N/A	

Study	Clinical area	Category	Outcomes/Measures	Subscale	Total outcomes examined
De Greef, 2011[73]	Diabetes	Biophysical	BMI	N/A	10
			FBG	N/A	
			HbA1c	N/A	
			tape measure cm (narrowest part of the torso)	N/A	
			total cholesterol	N/A	
		Health behavior	IPAQ (self-reported PA)	min/day housekeeping and gardening	
				min/day moderate-to-vigorous PA	
				min/day total PA	
				min/day walking during leisure time	
				steps/day	
D'Eramo Melkus, 2010[13]	Diabetes	Anxiety	psychosocial	PAID	25
		Biophysical	DSP	N/A	
			HbA1c	N/A	
			physiological	FBG	
				weight	
				LDL cholesterol	
				HDL cholesterol	
			SBP	N/A	
			TG	N/A	
		Health behavior	physiological	Current smoker	
		Pain	psychosocial	pain	
		Psychosocial	role-physical	N/A	
		Quality of life	psychosocial	QOL	
		Self-efficacy	psychosocial	diabetes self-efficacy	
		Functional status or disability	physical function	N/A	
		Health status	general health	N/A	
			vitality	N/A	
			mental health	somatic anxiety	
		Psychosocial	social function	N/A	
			role-emotional	N/A	
		Support	provider support	diet	
				exercise	
				knowledge	
				support	
Hornsten, 2008[17]	Diabetes	Biophysical	BMI	N/A	8
			DBP	N/A	
			HbA1c	N/A	
			HDL	N/A	
			LDL	N/A	
			SBP	N/A	
			total cholesterol	N/A	
			triglycerides	N/A	

Study	Clinical area	Category	Outcomes/Measures	Subscale	Total outcomes examined
Kulzer, 2007[72]	Diabetes	Anxiety	trait-anxiety symptoms	N/A	16
		Biophysical	BMI	N/A	
			cholesterol	N/A	
			FBG	N/A	
			HbA1c	N/A	
			HDL cholesterol	N/A	
			triglycerides	N/A	
			weight	weight	
		Health behavior	exercise	N/A	
			Three Factor Eating Questionnaire	cognitive restraint of eating	
				hunger	
				inhibition	
		Knowledge	diabetes knowledge	N/A	
		Self-efficacy	foot care	N/A	
			negative well-being	N/A	
			self care: urine or blood glucose self-test	N/A	
Lorig, 2009[69]	Diabetes	Anxiety/Depression	PHQ-9	N/A	17
		Biophysical	HbA1c	N/A	
			weight	N/A	
		Health behavior	aerobic exercise	N/A	
			communication with physician	N/A	
			glucose monitoring	N/A	
			healthy eating	N/A	
			read food labels	N/A	
		Health status	fatigue (VNS)	N/A	
			self-reported global health (NHS)	N/A	
			symptoms of hyperglycemia	N/A	
		Self efficacy	PAM	N/A	
			diabetes self-efficacy scale	N/A	
		Utilization	days in hospital	N/A	
			emergency visits	N/A	
			physician visits	N/A	
Lujan, 2007[78]	Diabetes	Biophysical	HbA1c (Bayer 2000 analyzer)	N/A	3
		Knowledge	DKQ (diabetes knowledge)	N/A	
		Self-efficacy	DHBM (diabetes health belief)	N/A	
Philis-Tsimikas, 2011[18]	Diabetes	Biophysical	BMI	N/A	8
			DBP	N/A	
			HbA1c	N/A	
			HDL	N/A	
			LDL	N/A	
			SBP	N/A	
			total cholesterol	N/A	
			triglycerides	N/A	
Raji, 2002[80]	Diabetes	Biophysical	BMI	N/A	2
			HbA1c	N/A	

Study	Clinical area	Category	Outcomes/Measures	Subscale	Total outcomes examined
Rickheim, 2002[74]	Diabetes	Attitudes	ATT-19 (psychosocial adjustment and attitudes towards diabetes)	N/A	10
		Biophysical	BMI	N/A	
			HbA1c	N/A	
			weight	N/A	
		Health behavior	exercise duration	N/A	
			exercise frequency	N/A	
		Knowledge	knowledge	N/A	
		Quality of life	SF-36	mental health	
				physical health	
		Self-efficacy	goal achieved	N/A	
Rosal, 2011[19]	Diabetes	Biophysical	BMI	N/A	19
			DBP	N/A	
			HbA1c	N/A	
			HDL cholesterol	N/A	
			LDL cholesterol	N/A	
			SBP	N/A	
			triglycerides	N/A	
			waist circumference	N/A	
		Health behavior	Alternative healthy eating index	N/A	
			sitting	N/A	
			total kcal	% fat	
				% SFA	
				% carbohydrates	
			total physical activity	N/A	
				duration	
			walking	N/A	
		Health status	Diabetes medication intensity score	N/A	
		Knowledge	Audit of Diabetes Knowledge	N/A	
		Self-efficacy	Study specific scale	diet and physical activity change	

Study	Clinical area	Category	Outcomes/Measures	Subscale	Total outcomes examined
Rygg, 2012[21]	Diabetes	Biophysical	BMI	N/A	22
			Creatinine	N/A	
			DBP	N/A	
			HbA1c	N/A	
			HDL	N/A	
			SBP	N/A	
			total cholesterol	N/A	
			triglycerides	N/A	
			weight	N/A	
		Knowledge	diabetes knowledge test	N/A	
		Psychosocial	PAID - problem areas in diabetes	N/A	
		Quality of life	EQ-5D (VAS)	N/A	
			SF-36	physical	
				mental health	
		Self-efficacy	PAM	N/A	
		Self-management	avoidance fatty foods	N/A	
			blood glucose monitoring	N/A	
			foot care	N/A	
			high vegetable intake	N/A	
		Treatment satisfaction	DTSQ	N/A	
		Utilization	medication (oral glucose lowering agents/insulin)	N/A	
			Utilization	N/A	
Sarkadi, 2004[81]	Diabetes	Biophysical	BMI	N/A	2
			HbA1c	N/A	
Scain, 2009[82]	Diabetes	Biophysical	BMI	N/A	10
			DBP	N/A	
			FBG	N/A	
			HbA1c	N/A	
			HDL cholesterol	N/A	
			SBP	N/A	
			total cholesterol	N/A	
			triglycerides	N/A	
			waist-hip ratio	N/A	
		Knowledge	knowledge	N/A	
Schillinger, 2009[30]	Diabetes	Biophysical	BMI	N/A	14
			DBP		
			HbA1c	NA	
			SBP		
		Functional status or disability	bed days	N/A	
			restricted activity	N/A	
		Health behavior	moderate physical activity	N/A	
			vigorous exercise	N/A	
		Quality of life	SF-12	physical health	
				mental health	
		Self-efficacy	behavioral	self-management	
			DQIP (diabetes self-efficacy)	NA	
			interpersonal processes of care	summary scale	
		Treatment satisfaction	patient assessment of chronic illness care	summary scale	

Study	Clinical area	Category	Outcomes/Measures	Subscale	Total outcomes examined
Sharifirad, 2012[83]	Diabetes	Biophysical	BMI	N/A	9
			DBP	N/A	
			HbA1C	N/A	
			HDL - cholesterol	N/A	
			LDL - cholesterol	N/A	
			SBP	N/A	
			triglycerides	N/A	
			weight	N/A	
			WHR	N/A	
Sperl-Hillen, 2011[84]	Diabetes	Anxiety/Depression	PAID (diabetes distress)	N/A	17
		Quality of life	SF-12	mental health	
				physical health	
		Biophysical	DBP	N/A	
			HbA1c	N/A	
			SBP	N/A	
			weight	N/A	
		Health behavior	BRFSS	physical activity score	
		Self-efficacy	RFS (food summary score)	N/A	
			DCP	care ability	
				importance of care	
				negative attitude	
				positive attitude	
				support attitudes	
				support received	
				understanding	
			DES-SF	N/A	
Steed, 2005[85]	Diabetes	Biophysical	HbA1c	N/A	20
		Health beliefs	beliefs	seriousness	
				treatment effectiveness	
				personal control	
		Knowledge	Knowledge	N/A	
		Mental health	HADS	mood	
			PANAS	negative affect	
				positive affect	
		Quality of life	ADDQOL	N/A	
			SF-36	N/A	
		Self-efficacy	MDS: multidimensional diabetes scale	total	
				diet	
				HBGM	
				exercise	
		Self-management	Revised summary of self care diabetes activities measure	N/A	
				diet	
				HBGM	
				foot care	
				smoking	

Study	Clinical area	Category	Outcomes/Measures	Subscale	Total outcomes examined
Toobert, 2011[86]	Diabetes	Biophysical	HbA1c	N/A	12
		Health behavior	% calories saturated fat	N/A	
			Chronic illness resources survey total score	N/A	
			physical activity (IPAQ)	N/A	
			smoking prevalence	N/A	
			stress management daily practice	N/A	
		Health status	UKPDS CHD	N/A	
		Problem solving ability	diabetes problem solving interview	N/A	
		Quality of life	CDC Healthy Days measure	physical health	
				mental health	
		Self-efficacy	COCSC	N/A	
		Social support	UCLA social support inventory	N/A	
Toobert, 2011[87]	Diabetes	Biophysical	HbA1c	N/A	10
		Health behavior	Chronic illness resources survey total score	N/A	
			stress management daily practice	N/A	
			% calories saturated fat	N/A	
			Physical activity (IPAQ)	N/A	
		Health status	UKPDS CHD	N/A	
		Problem solving ability	diabetes problem solving interview	N/A	
		Self-efficacy	COCSC	N/A	
		Biophysical	BMI	N/A	
		Social support	UCLA social support inventory	N/A	
Zapotozky, 2001[88]	Diabetes	Biophysical	Cholesterol	N/A	7
			DBP	N/A	
			HbA1c	N/A	
			HDL cholesterol	N/A	
			LDL cholesterol	N/A	
			SBP	N/A	
			triglycerides	N/A	
Surwit, 2002[20]	Diabetes	Anxiety	STAI	trait	8
				state	
		Anxiety/Depression	PSS	N/A	
		Biophysical	BMI	N/A	
			HbA1c	N/A	
		Health behavior	Dietary intake	N/A	
		Health status	DASI	N/A	
			GHQ	N/A	
Miller, 2002[79]	Diabetes	Biophysical	Fasting plasma glucose	N/A	6
			HbA1c	N/A	
			HDL cholesterol	N/A	
			LDL cholesterol	N/A	
			total cholesterol	N/A	
			triglycerides	N/A	

Study	Clinical area	Category	Outcomes/Measures	Subscale	Total outcomes examined
Smeulders, 2009[103] and 2010[27,60]	Heart failure	Anxiety/Depression	HADS	anxiety	21
				depression	
		Quality of life	RAND-36 and KCCQ	C-Qol sum score	
			RAND-36	G-QoL mental	
				G-QoL physical	
			KCCQ (cardiac-specific)	N/A	
		Self-efficacy	cognitive symptom management (Lorig et al. 1996)	N/A	
			EHFScBS	self-care behavior	
			perceived control (mastery scale by Pearlin and Schooler 1978)	N/A	
			VAS	perceived autonomy	
			GSES	general self-efficacy	
			two sub-scales CSEQ	cardiac self-efficacy	
			health behavior: drinking	N/A	
			health behavior: smoking	N/A	
		Functional status or disability	TICS (cognitive status)	N/A	
		Biophysical	BMI	N/A	
		Exercise tolerance	bicycling	N/A	
			other	N/A	
			swimming	N/A	
			walking	N/A	
		Utilization	number of MD and RN contacts	N/A	
Andryukhin, 2010[104]	Heart failure	Anxiety/Depression	HADS	anxiety	16
				depression	
		Biophysical	blood glucose	N/A	
			BMI	N/A	
			CRP	N/A	
			LASI	N/A	
			LDL	N/A	
			LVDVI	N/A	
			LVMI	N/A	
			NT-proBNP	N/A	
			total cholesterol	N/A	
		Exercise tolerance	6MWT	N/A	
			waist circumference	N/A	
		Quality of life	MLHFQ	emotional health	
				physical health	
				total level	
Chang, 2005[59]	Heart failure	Exercise tolerance	VO2max	N/A	5
		Quality of life	MLwHF	emotional health	
				physical health	
			peace and faith	N/A	
			strength (spiritual)	N/A	

Study	Clinical area	Category	Outcomes/Measures	Subscale	Total outcomes examined
Moore, 2006[58]	Heart failure	Anxiety/Depression	Depression/Dejection Scale	N/A	18
		Exercise tolerance	exercise amount	N/A	
			exercise frequency	N/A	
			exercise maintenance	N/A	
			6MWT	N/A	
		Functional status or disability	cardiac functional status	N/A	
			NYHA (cardiac functional status)	N/A	
		Pain	pain	N/A	
		Self-efficacy	benefits barriers: benefits	N/A	
			benefits barriers: barriers	N/A	
			benefits barriers: total	N/A	
			problem-solving inventory	N/A	
			total problem solving	N/A	
			self-efficacy: barriers	N/A	
			ASES (adherence)	N/A	
			ISR	N/A	
			SSES - social support	friends	
				family	
Nessman, 1980[62]	Hypertension	Self-efficacy	attendance	N/A	5
			pill count	N/A	
			test questions	N/A	
		Utilization	communications	N/A	
		Biophysical	blood pressure	N/A	
Rujiwatthanakorn, 2011[63]	Hypertension	Biophysical	BP diastolic	N/A	9
			BP systolic (Mate) (oscillometrics)	N/A	
		Exercise tolerance	SCABPCQ	self-care ability: aerobic exercise	
		Self-efficacy	KSCDQ	knowledge of self-care	
			SCABPCQ - self-care ability	dietary control	
				medication taking	
				risk behavior avoidance	
				self-monitoring	
				stress mgmt	
Baghianimoghadam, 2010[67]	Hypertension	Self-efficacy	Beliefs, Attitude, Subjective Norms, Enabling Factors (BASNEF) model	Attitude	5
				Subjective norms	
				Intention	
				Enabling factors	
				Self-monitoring	

Study	Clinical area	Category	Outcomes/Measures	Subscale	Total outcomes examined
Balcazar, 2009[64]	Hypertension	Anxiety	acculturative stress	N/A	14
			stress due to migration	N/A	
		Biophysical	BMI	N/A	
			waist circumference (inches)	N/A	
		Self-efficacy	family cohesiveness	N/A	
			Glindex score/acculturation	N/A	
			cholesterol and fat healthy habits	N/A	
			perceived barriers	N/A	
			perceived benefits	N/A	
			perceived severity	N/A	
			perceived susceptibility	N/A	
			salt and sodium healthy habits	N/A	
			self-efficacy	N/A	
			weight control healthy habits	N/A	
Burke, 2008[105]	Hypertension	Biophysical	blood lipids	N/A	26
			BMI	N/A	
			BP ambulatory	N/A	
			diastolic BP	N/A	
			glucose	N/A	
			HDL cholesterol	N/A	
			HOMA-IR (insulin)	N/A	
			insulin	N/A	
			systolic BP	N/A	
			total cholesterol	N/A	
			triglycerides	N/A	
		Exercise tolerance	physical activity	N/A	
		Self-efficacy	alcohol intake	N/A	
			calcium	N/A	
			diet	N/A	
			energy	N/A	
			fiber	N/A	
			magnesium	N/A	
			mono fat	N/A	
			poly fat	N/A	
			potassium	N/A	
			protein	N/A	
			sat fat intake	N/A	
			sodium	N/A	
			total fat	N/A	

Study	Clinical area	Category	Outcomes/Measures	Subscale	Total outcomes examined
Figar, 2006[65]	Hypertension	Biophysical	ABPM	day-time diastolic BP	11
				diastolic BP at program office	
				night-time diastolic BP	
				total diastolic BP	
			change in systolic BP	N/A	
			day-time systolic BP (6am-8pm)	N/A	
			night-time systolic BP (8:01 pm- 5:59am)	N/A	
			potassium excretion	N/A	
			sodium excretion	N/A	
			systolic BP at program office	N/A	
			total systolic BP	N/A	
Pierce, 1984[106]	Hypertension	Biophysical	BP reduction diastolic	N/A	6
			BP reduction systolic	N/A	
		Health status	clinician assessment	medication strength	
			clinician assessment	BP severity	
		Self-efficacy	daily monitoring	N/A	
			health education	N/A	
Scala, 2008[66]	Hypertension	Biophysical	DBP	N/A	7
			SBP	N/A	
		Exercise tolerance	daily physical activity	N/A	
		Self-efficacy	drug/alcohol/consumption	N/A	
			quantity of natural water consumption	N/A	
			salt intake	N/A	
			weight control	N/A	
Svetkey, 2009[26]	Hypertension	Biophysical	change in DBP	N/A	10
			change in SBP	N/A	
			FBG and lipids	N/A	
			urinary sodium	N/A	
			weight	N/A	
		Exercise tolerance	physical activity	N/A	
		Self-efficacy	dairy (servings/day)	N/A	
			dietary pattern	N/A	
			sat fat	N/A	
			total fat	N/A	
Clemson, 2004[24]	History of falls	Anxiety	Worry scale	N/A	7
		Functional status or disability	PASE (physical activity)	N/A	
		Quality of life	SF-36	mental health	
				physical health	
		Self-efficacy	mobility efficacy scale (MES)	falls	
			modified falls efficacy scale (MFES)	falls	
			FaB scale (behaviors fall prevention)	N/A	

Study	Clinical area	Category	Outcomes/Measures	Subscale	Total outcomes examined
Arnold, 2008[107]	History of falls	Falls	falls-efficacy	N/A	9
		Physical performance	(hip abduction strength)	N/A	
			6MWT (gait)	N/A	
			BBSm (balance)	N/A	
			lower body strength	N/A	
			max step length	N/A	
			MCTSIB (balance function)	N/A	
			ROM (hip flexion range of motion)	N/A	
			TUG (mobility)	N/A	
Shumway-Cook, 2007[25]	History of falls	Falls	fall incidence rates	N/A	4
		Functional status or disability	mobility	N/A	
		Physical performance	balance	N/A	
			strength	N/A	
Arnold, 2010[45]	History of falls	Falls efficacy	ABC (balance)	N/A	7
		Functional status or disability	AIMS-2 (daily function)	N/A	
			PASE (physical activity)	N/A	
		Physical performance	6MWT	N/A	
			BBS (balance)	N/A	
			chair stands	N/A	
			TUG (mobility)	N/A	
Ryan, 1996[46]	History of falls	Falls	N fall events including descriptions	N/A	3
			N fall prevention changes implemented	N/A	
			type of fall prevention changes made	N/A	
Ersek, 2003[97]	Pain	Anxiety/Depression	GDS	N/A	8
		Functional status or disability	SF-36	physical functioning	
				role-physical	
		Pain	GCPS	pain intensity	
				related activity interference	
			SOPA	pain-related beliefs-SOPA control	
				pain-related beliefs-SOPA harm	
				pain-related beliefs-SOPA medical care	
Vlaeyen, 1996[96]	Pain	Anxiety	FSS-III-R (fear)	N/A	12
			PCL, CSQ (catastrophizing)	N/A	
		Anxiety/Depression	BDI	N/A	
		Health status	MOCI (obsessive-compulsive)	N/A	
		Pain	BAT (activity)	N/A	
			CSQ	relaxation	
				pain coping	
			CSQ, MPLC	pain control	
			MPQ (pain intensity)	N/A	
			UAB, CHIP, BAT (pain behavior)	N/A	
		Quality of life/Pain	tension	N/A	
		Self-efficacy	knowledge	N/A	

Study	Clinical area	Category	Outcomes/Measures	Subscale	Total outcomes examined
Gustavsson, 2010[98]	Pain	Anxiety	CSQ	catastrophizing	14
			FABQ fear (work place)	N/A	
			HADS	anxiety	
		Anxiety/Depression	HADS	depression	
		Functional status or disability	NDI (neck disability)	N/A	
		Pain	NDI (analgesics due to neck pain)	N/A	
			VAS	average (pain scale)	
				present (pain scale)	
				worst (pain scale)	
		Self-efficacy	CSQ	ability to control pain	
				ability to reduce pain	
				N/A	
			SES	N/A	
		Utilization	satisfaction with care/treatment (5-pt scale)	N/A	
Haugli, 2003[95]	Pain	Anxiety/Depression	General Health Questionnaire (GHQ)	psychological distress	4
		Health status	GHQ	group status	
				sick leave	
			days absent due to pain (last 6 mo)	N/A	
		Pain	VAS	pain	
				pain coping	
		Self-efficacy	VAS	management of daily life	

APPENDIX D. PEER REVIEW COMMENTS AND RESPONSES

Reviewer	Comment	Response
Q1. Are the objectives, scope, and methods for this review clearly described?		
1	Yes. (No comment)	Noted.
2	Yes. (No comment)	Noted.
3	Yes. (No comment)	Noted.
4	Yes. (No comment)	Noted.
5	Yes. Detailed table of contents. Objectives are listed in the Executive Summary under the background information.	Noted.
6	Yes. (No comment)	Noted.
7	Yes. There was not really enough evidence but perhaps a weakness is that the groups run by peers and professionals could not be separated	Noted.
8	Yes. (No comment)	Noted.
9	Yes. Absolutely, very inclusive	Noted.
10	Yes. (No comment)	Noted.
Q2. Is there any indication of bias in our synthesis of the evidence?		
1	No. No evidence for bias.	Noted.
2	No. (No comment)	Noted.
3	No. (No comment)	Noted.
4	No. (No comment)	Noted.
5	No. I felt that the review utilized a variety of databases to obtain a large number of articles related to group visits. Some of the studies looked at were done within the VA but in my opinion, the review did not provide any type of bias.	Noted.
6	No. (No comment)	Noted.
7	No. (No comment)	Noted.
8	No. (No comment)	Noted.
9	No, it was excellent	Noted.
10	No. (No comment)	Noted.
Q3. Are the objectives, scope, and methods for this review clearly described?		
1	No. I am not aware of overlooked data sources.	Noted.
2	No. (No comment)	Noted.

Group Visits Focusing on Education for the Management of Chronic Conditions in Adults

Reviewer	Comment	Response
3	Yes. Much of my focus has been intervention on blood pressure control in the group session, so some of the studies mentioned below have a slant towards treating hypertension.	Two of the suggested papers (Cakir, Saounatsu) were a combination of group and individual visits, and it was impossible to separate out the effects of these respective intervention components. We examined the Palomaki study and decided against including it because the study design was not a randomized controlled trial.
	Appel, L.J., Chanpagne,C.M., Harsha, D.W., Cooper, L.S., Obarzanek, E., Elmer, P.J., Stevens, V.J, W.M., P. H., Svetkey, L.P., Stedman, S.W., Young, D.R., and Writing Group of the Premier Collaborative Research Group. 2003. Effects of comprehensive lifestyle modification on blood pressure control: main results of the Premier clinical trial. JAMA. 289:2083-2093	
	Baghianimoghadam, M.H., Rahaee, Z., Morowatisharifabad, M.A., Sharifrad, G., Andishmand, A., and Azadbakht, L. 2010. Effects of education on self monitoring of blood pressure based on BASNEF model in hypertensive patients. J RES MED SCI. 15:70-77	We agree that the Baghianimoghadam study should be included, which we have done, and have amended our results accordingly.
	Cakir, H., and Pinar, R. 2006. Randomized controlled trial on lifestyle modification in hypertensive patients…including commentary by: Clark AM and response by Pinar and Cakir. West.J.Nurs.Res.28: 190-215	We cited the Appel paper in the Limitation section as an example of a good quality study that combined group and individual visits without analyzing the group visit component separately, and clarified that we did not include these studies.
	Palomaki, A., Miilunpalo, S., Holm, P., Makinen, E., and Malminiem, L. 2002 Effects of preventive group education on the resistance of LDL against oxidation and risk factors for coronary heart disease in bypass surgery patients. ANN.Med. 34:272-283	
	Saounatsou, M., Patsi, O., Fasoi, G., Stylianou, M., Kavga, A., Economou, O., Mandi, P., and Nicolaou, M. 2001. The influence of the hypertensive patient's education in compliance with their medication. Public Health Nurs. 18:436-442	
4	No. (No comment)	Noted.
5	No. Not that I am aware of.	Noted.
6	No. (No comment)	Noted.
7	Yes. Kearns, J.W. et al (2012) Group diabetes education administered through telemedicine: Tools used and lessons learned. Telemedicine and EHealth, 18, p347.	We examined the suggested study and decided against including it because the study design was not a randomized controlled trial.
8	None of which I am aware	Noted.
9	No. Have you looked at the shared medical appointment esp or the realist review of evidence synthesis for shared medical appointments	We thank the reviewer for the suggestion. Yes, we have examined the shared medical appointment (SMA) ESP report and have noted that these reports are complementary reviews of group appointments. In addition, we developed our library in collaboration with the SMA group to ensure that there was no overlap in the included literature.
10	No. (No comment)	Noted.

Group Visits Focusing on Education for the Management of Chronic Conditions in Adults

Evidence-based Synthesis Program

Q4. Please write additional suggestions or comments below. If applicable, please indicate the page and line numbers from the draft report.

Reviewer	Comment	Response
2	Page 10, last sentence-examples given of "non-prescribing providers only include "nurses and nurse educators" Although other disciplines are listed later, expanding the variety of disciplines in this sentence may more clearly show that it is not just a nurse-run group visit.	We have expanded the list of examples given on pg. 10, per the reviewer's suggestion.
3	I must say I was disappointed that the great majority of studies fail to show a preponderance of evidence for the efficacy of the group medical experience versus standard treatment options in primary care, at least in the short-term. It appears that many studies showed some improvement in certain aspects such as blood pressure readings or a reduction in LDL numbers, but not very much evidence for long-term gains in overall physical health. It doesn't appear that there are enough studies done in a longitudinal fashion that would lend themselves to basing any conclusions of long-term gains. Being someone who believes in the group experience for patients, and who is continuing to use them in the form of drop in group medical appointments, or shared medical appointments under a heading of hypertension or diabetes, I was hoping for more evidence that would point to increasing the use of these types of clinic experiences.	We thank the reviewer for the thoughtful comments. We agree that there is a need for trials that evaluate outcomes over longer periods of time, and the utility of booster sessions. We have noted these gaps in the evidence base in the Future Research section.
6	The review is very well written, including the Generalizability and Limitations sections. Page 60, last sentence, remove "the", "...to attend a multi-week course" ...	We thank the reviewer for the feedback on the readability of the report, and have made the suggested change.
8	In the last sentence on page 10 (Introduction Section), the report states, "This review...focuses exclusively on literature that tests the effectiveness of group visits that have an emphasis on health education and are led by **non-prescribing providers** such as nurses and nurse educators." It is my understanding that the intent of the report is to review studies in which the group visits are led by non-prescribing health professionals (e.g., nurses, dietitians). Given this, should those studies described in the "Multiple Chronic Conditions" section (page 59) be included in this review since all but the Elzen (2007) study were led by peer leaders and not health care professionals?	We have included trials of group visits led by peer educators as well as social workers, and believe this is an important aspect to many group visit interventions that ought to be represented in the report. As a complement to the shared medical appointment report, this review was intended to expand the purview of group appointment interventions to include those led by personnel that are non-physicians. We have clarified that we include group visit facilitators that exclude prescribing providers and may include health professionals (e.g., nurses, dietitians, physical therapists).
8	The recently released report on Shared Medical Appointments included a table in the "Future Research Section" that identified evidence gaps and suggested types of studies to close those gaps. Would it be possible to include a similar table in this report?	Yes, we agree that the Future Research section in table form, similar to the one used in the shared medical appointments report, is a useful way to display gaps in the research done in this area. We have made this change.

Reviewer	Comment	Response
9	This is definitely a contribution. I hope that in the discussion that you may add that areas that demonstrate some benefit but the studies are not strong, may be areas for further pilot testing in the field with more data collecting. I don't personally believe that the only answer is more rigorous studies, but more practice with the evidence we have. Patients' self efficacy and satisfaction with chronic disease care is critical for VA in the future when veterans can choose where they get their healthcare. Low cost options that may improve even short term outcomes may be worth investing in, especially when led by peers and in the community. I don't want to discourage that type of clinical care. Happy to talk further. Would be happy to be involved in writing a paper about this and comparing to sma ESP and sma realist review.	We thank the reviewer for the thoughtful comments. We have added suggestions for further pilot testing in the field and more efforts for data collection to the Future Research section.
10	Here are some minor modifications. 1) Changes to Group Visits Draft: Use of "dietitian" on pages 12, 47, 49, 86 – please spell with a "t" instead of a "c" in dietician 2) In Generalizability section, last sentence- p. , suggest use of terminology "who demonstrated motivation " instead of "who have enough motivation" which appears vague 3) Limitations p. 71- "Knowledge improvement outcomes" instead of "knowledge outcomes" even if knowledge was not studied, the use of knowledge does not indicate any qualitative or quantitative changes	Noted. We have made these changes.

Q5. Are there any VA clinical performance measures, programs, quality improvement measures, patient care services, or conferences that will be directly affected by this report? If so, please provide detail.

Reviewer	Comment	Response
1	Yes. Current primary care clinical performance is evaluated on percentage of encounters that are done in group setting, including educational and self management groups offered by nursing and other staff. I expect this will impact what conditions are treated in this fashion, with self-management preferred over didactic methods.	Noted.
2	Not directly by this report but this report in conjunction with the SMA report from Durham may have an impact on SMAs in PACT. Could influence targets in Compass related to non-single provider face-to-face visits in PACT.	Noted.
3	Yes—there is certainly a "push" within the VA for expansion of the use of group medical appointments and shared medical appointments. Some of the focus in PACT (Patient Aligned Care Teams) within the VA is the use by the care team in fashioning unique and "out of the box" alternatives to the usual one patient-one provider-one visit model. There has also been a focus on applying evidence based practice measures to our daily practice in hopes of improving patient care. The VA will have to continue to look at group medical experiences, and the research that is available to determine how much emphasis is placed on the utilization of these particular experiences, as well as looking at the long term effects of these types of encounters to ascertain long-term benefit.	Noted.

Reviewer	Comment	Response
5	Group visits are listed under Access in the 2012 Compass Goals for VISN 12. Currently, groups are available for diabetes, lipids, CHF, and weight management. To meet access goals, groups allow more veterans to be seen in a timely manner. Individual appointment are also available, groups are not exclusive.	Noted.
6	Not aware.	Noted.
7	Many sites are implementing group education to meet performance measures for DM	Noted.
8	Given that VHA has prioritized group visits as part of the new primary care model, staff who are members of PACT teams will be directly affected by this report. There are currently VA facilities where nurses are involved in group visits. In the next couple of weeks, the Office of Nursing Services, through the ONS liaisons to PACT and Specialty Care, will attempt to obtain a list of the sites that currently conduct group visits along with the target population for those group visits. Additionally, the national Diabetes Program, the national Pain Program, and the National Center for Patient Safety (falls) would likely be interested in this report.	Noted.
9	This is a part of PACT and NCP. We can disseminate findings through them at a national level. Michael Goldstein and Margaret Dundon.	Noted.

Q6. Please provide any recommendations on how this report can be revised to more directly address or assist implementation needs.

1	It would be helpful to have data about what VA's are currently offering in relation to these conditions.	We agree that it would be helpful to discuss implementation of group visits and shared medical appointments within the context of what the VA currently offers for Veterans with chronic conditions. Although these considerations are important, this discussion extends beyond the scope of this review.
2	It would be helpful to not only know whether group visits affects the usage/frequency of traditional care but whether the traditional visit is altered when patients also attend group visits. For example, is the focus of the single provider face-to-face visit changed when patients also attend group visits (ie. patients that attend pain SMAs may still see their provider on the same schedule but they may be able to address more issues unrelated to pain whereas in the past the majority of the visit focused on pain-related issues).	This is a very interesting point. It would be an interesting premise for additional qualitative studies examining the quality of care provided in GVs as a complement to traditional individual clinical visits. We included studies of comparative effectiveness of head-to-head individual visits versus group visits. Unfortunately, there were few of these studies and we have identified this as a gap in the research base in the Future Research section.

Group Visits Focusing on Education for the Management of Chronic Conditions in Adults

Reviewer	Comment	Response
3	Happily the research does not seem to be saying that there is not benefit to the group experiences, but it does seem to point to the issue of perhaps longer studies being necessary. Also, how a patient perceives benefit from a group experience whether the data seems to show an actual "health benefit "is a much more nebulous and decidedly more difficult factor to measure. The VA will have to be prudent in using group experiences so that the focus continues to be looking to research to guide implementation of these appointments versus using these because of fiscal concerns.	We agree with the reviewer and have made these points in the Future Research and Discussion sections.
5	Cost and specifically Medicare reimbursement have been the driving forces for group education in the private sector. In the VA, however, group education has been a means to improving better access—see more veterans in a timely manner. I am curious to know if length of class time (60, 90, 120min) or number of group visits(3-12 sessions) negatively influenced the group findings related to the 3 key questions? Individual visits might have been shorter (30-60 minutes) and only required 1 or 2 visits. Ultimately giving patients a choice in how they receive education—individual vs. group—is patient centric. A synthesized review showing that the results appear to be similar whether they receive individual or group education seem to support this new health care philosophy. I would encourage more research in the area of secured messaging and how that use of technology might affect patient outcomes in the management of chronic diseases. I would also encourage research in the area of MOVE! Groups and how they compare to individual visits.	We abstracted length and duration of group visits in the expectation that we would be able to compare trials based on these important elements. However, heterogeneity between trials was significant and precluded examination of these important questions. We agree that further research is needed and have identified various gaps in the Future Research section that the reviewer also identifies.
6	As a geriatrician, my concern is that somewhat positive findings from RCTs of group appointments may not necessarily translate into improved outcomes in real life situation, given the selection bias inherent to characteristics of research participants in general (usually more motivated and concerned about their health). I just read a study from Netherlands that looked at older individuals' preferences for educational programs on falls and found that the majority (62.7%) had no interest to participate in any format; in addition, poor perceived health and age over 80 were associated with less preference for a group program format. (Dorresteijn, TA, Rixt Zijlstra GA, Van Eijs YJ, Vlaeyen JW, Kempen GI. Older people's preferences regarding programme formats for managing concerns about falls. Age Aging . 2012;41(4):474-81) It seems that given the weak evidence and the heterogeneity of intervention content and outcomes, the implementation of group appointments, especially in Geri PACTs, should not be rushed, because having to come in for a group appointment may not be the "most patient centered care" for a frail older individual. Also, additional evaluations should be incorporated early on, in this VHA implementation effort, so that meaningful conclusions could be made in the future on the value of group appointments in the VA.	The reviewer brings up some very important and interesting considerations. Although we did not find any direct harms, the VA should be cautious given the lack of robust findings that GV improve health outcomes. In addition, there is potential for downsides to GV implementation. For example, travel time involved to get to and participate in GVs, which as the reviewer points out, may be a salient and prohibitive factor for frail, older participants. Given the relatively low benefits in health outcomes and the risk of inconvenience, we need to be careful about making blanket recommendations of group visits, particularly for patient populations with specific health needs. We have included these points in the Discussion section.
9	National PACT calls or community of practice	Noted.

Group Visits Focusing on Education for the Management of Chronic Conditions in Adults

Reviewer	Comment	Response
Q7. Please provide us with contact details of any additional individuals/stakeholders who should be made aware of this report.		
1	Primary Care leadership, Mental Health leadership	Noted.
2	Susan Kirsh, Sharon Watts	Noted.
6	VACO GEC	Noted.
7	PACT and Specialty care clinical teams will benefit HRSD should be aware of this as there is a gap in knowledge	Noted.
8	As soon as the ESP program knows the date of the CyberSeminar when this report will be released, could you please send this information to Bev Priefer in the Office of Nursing Services so that we can do some advance notification of the various nursing groups that will be interested in this report.	Noted.
9	Dr stark, dr schectman, me, dr kinsinger, dr Goldstein, ONS, Anthony morreale in pharmacy	Noted.
10	Additional stakeholders include Primary Care Leaders to share with PACT teamlets and teams, and MOVE! Coordinators. The PACT and ACCESS goals promote the use of group education to manage chronic diseases. Additionally, individual visits are still available, offering Veteran's a choice.	Noted.

Return to Contents

APPENDIX E. GLOSSARY FOR OUTCOMES USED IN INCLUDED STUDIES

Acronym	Measure/Outcome
28 JC	28 Joint Count
AAMP	Australian Asthma Management Plan
AASA	Asthma Attitude Survey for Adults (24-item)
ABC	Activities-specific Balance Confidence
ABPM	Ambulatory Blood Pressure Monitoring
ADAPT	Arthritis, diet and physical activity promotion trial
ADDQOL	Audit of Diabetes-Dependent Quality of Life
AGKQ	Asthma General Knowledge Questionnaire
AHI	Arthritis Helplessness Index
AIMS2/Dutch-AIMS2	Arthritis Impact Measurement Scales version 2
AIMS2: AS	Arthritis Impact Measurement Scales version 2: Affect Subscale
AIMS2: CHS	Arthritis Impact Measurement Scales version 2: Current Health Subscale
AIMS2: PFS	Arthritis Impact Measurement Scales version 2: Physical Function Subscale
AIMS2: SS	Arthritis Impact Measurement Scales version 2: Symptom Subscale
ANCOVA	Analysis of Covariance
AQLQ	Asthma Quality of Life Questionnaire
AQOL	Assessment of Quality of Life
ASCQ	Arthritis Stages of Change
ASES	Asthma or Arthritis Self-efficacy Scale
ASMP	Arthritis Self-Management Program
BAI	Beck Anxiety Inventory
BASNEF	Belief, Attitude, Subjective Norm, Enabling Factors educational model
BAT	Behavioral Approach Test
BDI and BDI-II	Beck Depression Inventory
BIQ	Basic Information Quiz (51-item)
BMI	Body Mass Index
BRFSS	Behavioral Risk Factor Surveillance System
CBT	Cognitive Behavioral Therapy
CCQ	Clinical COPD Questionnaire
CES-D	Center for Epidemiologic Studies Depression Scale
CHANGE	Change Habits by Applying New Goals and Experiences
CHIP	Checklist for Interpersonal Pain Behavior
COCSC	Confidence in Overcoming Challenges to Self-Care instrument
COPE	Community-based physiotherapeutic exercise program
CORS	Coping With Rheumatoid Stressors
CQ	Asthma Knowledge Questionnaire (12-item)
CRDQ (aka CRQ)	Chronic Respiratory Disease Questionnaire
CRQ-SAS	Chronic Respiratory Questionnaire Standardised

Acronym	Measure/Outcome
CSEQ	Cardiac Self-efficacy Questionnaire (two sub-scales)
DAS28	Disease Activity Score using 28 joint counts
DASI	Duke Activity Status Index
DCP	Diabetes Care Profile
DES-SF	Diabetes Empowerment Scale, Short Form
DHBM	Diabetes Health Belief Measure
DKQ	Diabetes Knowledge Questionnaire
DQIP	Diabetes Quality Improvement Program
DSMP	Diabetes Self-management Program
DTSQ	Diabetes Treatment Satisfaction Questionnaire
EADL	Extended Activities of Daily Living
EMIR	French Quality of Life of RA (using short version of AIMS2-SF)
EMS	Early Morning Joint Stiffness
EQ-5D: VAS	Five Dimensional Health State Description of EuroQol
ESR	Erythrocyte Sedimentation Rate
ESWT	Endurance Shuttle Walk Test
EURIDISS	EUropean Research on Incapacitating Diseases and Social Support
EuroQol	Euro Quality of Life
FaB scale	Falls Behavioural Scale (behaviors protective of falls)
FABQ	Fear Avoidance Belief Questionnaire
FACIT-F	Functional Assessment of Chronic Illness Therapy-Fatigue
FAST	Fitness Arthritis and Senior Trial
FBG	Fasting Blood Glucose
FEV	Forced Expiratory Volume
FFM	Percentage of Fat Free Mass
FIT	Educational and physical training program
FPI	Functional Performance Inventory
FSS-III-R	Distinguishes 5 types of fears/phobias
GCPS	Chronic Pain Scale
GDS	Geriatric Depression Scale
GHQ	General Health Questionnaire
GSES-16	General Self-Efficacy Scale
GV	Group visit
HAAS	Hypothetical Asthma Attack Scenarios
HADS	Hospital Anxiety and Depression Scale
HAQ	Health Assessment Questionnaire
heiQ	Health Education Impact Questionnaire
HJAM	Hand Joint Alignment and Motion Scale
HJC	Hand Joint Count
HOMA-IR	Homeostasis Model Assessment of Insulin Resistance

Acronym	Measure/Outcome
HRQOL	Health-related Quality of Life
HSI	Heaviness of Smoking Index
IDEA	Interactive Dialogue to Educate and Activate
IDEALL	Improving Diabetes Efforts Across Language and Literacy
IPAQ	International Physical Activity Questionnaire
IPQ-R	Revised Illness Perceptions Questionnaire
ISR	Index of Self-Religion
ISWT	Incremental Shuttle Walk Test
JP	Joint Protection
JPBA	Joint Protection Behavior Assessment
JPKA	Joint Protection Knowledge Assessment
K10	Kessler Psychological Distress Scale
KCCQ	Kansas City Cardiomyopathy Questionnaire
KSCDQ	Knowledge of Self-Care Demands Questionnaire
LASI	Left Atrial Size Index
LMAP	Lifestyle management for arthritis programme
LVDVI	LV Diastolic Volume Index
LVMI	Left Ventricular Mass Index
MAF	Multidimensional Assessment of Fatigue Scale
MAPT	Multi-Attribute Prioritisation Tool
MARS	Medication Adherence Report Scale (5-item)
mCTSIB	Modified Clinical Test of Sensory Interaction on Balance
MDS	Multidimensional Diabetes Scale
M-HAQ	Mobility-Health Assessment Questionnaire
MLHFQ (aka MLwHF)	Minnesota Living With Heart Failure
MOCI	Maudsley Obsessive-Compulsive Inventory
MOS	Medical Outcomes Survey (measures of quality of life core survey)
MPLC	Multidimensional Pain Locus of Control Scale
MPQ	McGill Pain Questionnaire
MRC	Medical Research Council
NDI	Neck Disability Index
NHP	Nottingham Health Profile
NT-proBNP	N-terminal pro-brain natriuretic peptide
NYHA	New York Heart Association Classification
OT	Occupational therapist
PAID	Problem Areas in Diabetes Survey
PAM	Patient Activation Measure
PANAS	Positive and Negative Affect Schedule
PASE	Physical Activity Scale for the Elderly
PASS	Pain and stress self-management program

Acronym	Measure/Outcome
PCL	Pain Cognition List
PEF	Peak Expiratory Flow
PEM	Self-management empowerment education model
PIHAQ	Personal Impact Health Assessment Questionnaire
PSS	Perceived Stress Scale
PT	Physical therapist
QALYs	Stanford Health Assessment Questionnaire
QOL	Quality of life
RAI: AHS	Rheumatology Attitudes Index: Arthritis Helplessness Subscale
RAI: AIS	Rheumatology Attitudes Index: Arthritis Internality Subscale
RAND-36	RAND 36-Item Health Survey
RAQol	Rheumatoid Arthritis Quality of Life
RASE	RA Self-efficacy
RFS	Food Summary Score
ROM	Range of Motion
SCABPCQ	Self-Care Ability for Blood Pressure Control Questionnaire
SES	Self-efficacy Scale
SF-12	The 12-Item Short Form Health Survey
SF-36	Short Form Health Survey
SGRQ	St. George's Respiratory Questionnaire
SMART	Self-management arthritis relief therapy
SOPA	Survey of Pain Attitudes
SPSMQ	Short Portable Mental Status Questionnaire
SSAI	State Anxiety Inventory
SSES	Strengths Self-Efficacy Scale
STAI	Spielberger State-Trait Anxiety Inventory
TFEQ	Three Factor Eating Questionnaire
TICS	Telephone Interview for Cognitive Status
TSES	Total Self-efficacy Scale
TUG	Timed Up and Go
UAB	Pain Behavior Scale
UCL-DSMP	University College London-Diabetes Self-management Program
VAS	Visual Analog Scale
VNS	Visual Numeric Scale for pain (modified VAS)
VO2max	Maximal Oxygen Uptake
WHOQOL-BREF	World Health Organization quality of life instrument, short version
WOMAC	Western Ontario and McMaster Universities Osteoarthritis

www.ingramcontent.com/pod-product-compliance
Lightning Source LLC
Chambersburg PA
CBHW081728170526
45167CB00009B/3744